This book is due for return on or before the last date shown below.

Evidence-Based Practice

Guest Editor

ALYCE A. SCHULTZ, RN, PhD, FAAN

NURSING CLINICS OF NORTH AMERICA

www.nursing.theclinics.com

Consulting Editor
SUZANNE S. PREVOST, RN, PhD, COI

March 2009 • Volume 44 • Number 1

SAUNDERS an imprint of ELSEVIER, Inc.

W.B. SAUNDERS COMPANY

A Division of Elsevier Inc.

1600 John F. Kennedy Blvd., Suite 1800 ● Philadelphia, PA 19103-2899

http://www.theclinics.com

NURSING CLINICS OF NORTH AMERICA Volume 44, Number 1
March 2009 ISSN 0029-6465, ISBN-13: 978-1-4377-0508-9, ISBN-10: 1-4377-0508-1

Editor: Katie Hartner
Developmental Editor: Theresa Collier

Nursing Clinics of North America (ISSN 0029-6465) is published quarterly by Elsevier Inc., 360 Park Avenue South, New York, NY 10010-1710. Months of issue are March, June, September, and December. Business and Editorial Offices: 1600 John F. Kennedy Blvd., Suite 1800, Philadelphia, PA 19103-2899. Periodicals postage paid at New York, NY and additional mailing offices. Subscription price per year is, $133.00 (US individuals), $273.00 (US institutions), $228.00 (international individuals), $334.00 (international institutions), $184.00 (Canadian individuals), $334.00 (Canadian institutions), $70.00 (US students), and $115.00 (international students). To receive student/resident rate, orders must be accompanied by name of affiliated institution, date of term, and the signature of program/residency coordinator on institution letterhead. Orders will be billed at individual rate until proof of status is received. Foreign air speed delivery is included in all *Clinics* subscription prices. All prices are subject to change without notice. **POSTMASTER:** Send address changes to *Nursing Clinics*, Elsevier Periodicals Customer Service, 11830 Westline Industrial Drive, St. Louis, MO 63146. **Customer Service: 1-800-654-2452 (US). From outside the United States, call 1-314-453-7041. Fax: 1-314-453-5170. E-mail: JournalsCustomerService-usa@elsevier.com** (for print support) and **JournalsOnlineSupport-usa @elsevier.com** (for online support).

Nursing Clinics of North America is covered in EMBASE/Excerpta Medica, MEDLINE/PubMed (Index Medicus), Social Sciences Citation Index, Current Contents, ASCA, Cumulative Index to Nursing, RNdex Top 100, and Allied Health Literature and International Nursing Index (INI).

Printed in the United States of America.

Contributors

CONSULTING EDITOR

SUZANNE S. PREVOST, RN, PhD, COI
Associate Dean, Practice and Community Engagement, University of Kentucky, Lexington, Kentucky

GUEST EDITOR

ALYCE A. SCHULTZ, RN, PhD, FAAN
President, EBP Concepts, Alyce A. Schultz & Associates, LLC, Chandler, Arizona

AUTHORS

REBECCA ALLEGRETTO, RN, BSN
Clinical Nurse Coordinator, Thoracic Surgery, Ronald Reagan University of California Los Angeles Medical Center, Los Angeles, California

JACQUELINE J. ANDERSON, MSN, RN
Director, Nursing Programs Quality, Division of Nursing, The University of Texas MD Anderson Cancer Center, Houston, Texas; and Former Director, Nursing Research, St. Luke's Episcopal Hospital, Houston, Texas

RENEE APPLEBY, RN
Unit Director, Cardiothoracic Surgery Unit, Department of Nursing, Ronald Reagan University of California Los Angeles Medical Center, Los Angeles, California

JAQUELINE M. ATTLESEY-PRIES, MS, RN
Nurse Administrator, Nursing Practice Resource Division, Department of Nursing, Mayo Clinic Rochester, Rochester, Minnesota

KAREN BALAKAS, PhD, RN, CNE
Associate Professor, Goldfarb School of Nursing at Barnes-Jewish College, St. Louis, Missouri

DORA BRADLEY, PhD, RN-BC
Vice President, Nursing Professional Development, Baylor Health Care System, Corporate Office of Chief Nursing Officer, Dallas, Texas

KATHERINE BRADY-SCHLUTTNER, MS, RN-BC
Nursing Education Specialist and Assistant Professor, Education and Professional Development Division, Department of Nursing, Mayo Clinic Rochester, Rochester, Minnesota

BARBARA B. BREWER, PhD, RN, MALS, MBA
Director of Professional Practice, John C. Lincoln North Mountain Hospital, Phoenix, Arizona

MELANIE A. BREWER, DNSc, RN, FNP-BC
Director, Nursing Research, Scottsdale Healthcare, Scottsdale, Arizona

M. KATHLEEN BREWER, PhD, ARNP, BC
Associate Professor, University of Kansas School of Nursing, Kansas City, Kansas

KAREN BURKETT, MS, RN, CNP
Evidence-Based Practice Mentor, Center for Professional Excellence-Research and Evidence-Based Practice, Cincinnati Children's Hospital Medical Center, Cincinnati, Ohio

PAULETTE BURNS, PhD, RN
Dean, Harris College of Nursing and Health Sciences, Texas Christian University, Fort Worth, Texas

SUE CULLEN, RN, MSN
Director of Education, Education Department, Acadia Hospital, Bangor, Maine

JOHN F. DIXON, MSN, RN, CNA, BC
Nurse Researcher and Interim Director, BUMC Center for Nursing Education and Research, Baylor University Medical Center, Dallas, Texas

SUE ELLIS-HERMANSEN, RN, MS
President, Omicron Xi Chapter At-Large, Sigma Theta Tau International Honor Society; and Director of Learning Resource Center/Lecturer, School of Nursing, University of Maine, Orono, Maine

DOREEN K. FRUSTI, MSN, MS, RN
Chair, Department of Nursing; and Co-Director, NQF Scholars Program, Department of Nursing, Mayo Clinic Rochester, Rochester, Minnesota

PAULETTE GALLANT, RN, MSN, CNL
Clinical Nurse Leader, Maine Medical Center, Portland, Maine

ANNA GAWLINSKI, RN, DNSc, CS-ACNP
Director of Evidence-Based Practice, Department of Nursing, Ronald Reagan University of California Los Angeles Medical Center; and Adjunct Professor, University of California Los Angeles School of Nursing, Los Angeles, California

MARCELLINE R. HARRIS, PhD, RN
Nurse Administrator/Nurse Researcher, NQF Scholars Program Director, Division of Nursing Informatics and Nursing Health Sciences Research, Department of Nursing, Mayo Clinic Rochester, Rochester, Minnesota

BARBARA HIGGINS, RNC, PhD
Chair of Nursing, Department of Nursing, Husson College, Bangor, Maine

CYNTHIA HONESS, RN, MSN, CCRN, ACNS-BC
Cardiology Clinical Nurse Specialist, Center for Clinical and Professional Development, Department of Nursing, Maine Medical Center, Portland, Maine

KATHLEEN KEANE, RN BSN, CCRN
Clinical Nurse II, Cardiothoracic Intensive Care Unit, Maine Medical Center, Portland, Maine

KELLY LANCASTER, RN, BSN, CAPA
Maine Medical Center, Scarborough Surgery Center, Scarborough, Maine

PHYLLIS LAWLOR-KLEAN, RNC, MS, APN/CNS
Advanced Practice Nurse, Neonatal Intensive Care Unit, Advocate Christ Medical
Center/Hope Children's Hospital, Oak Lawn, Illinois

CHERYL A. LEFAIVER, PhD, RN
Professional Nurse Researcher, Advocate Christ Medical Center/Hope Children's
Hospital, Oak Lawn, Illinois

CHERYL N. LINDY, PhD, RN-BC, NEA-BC
Director, Nursing and Patient Education and Research; and Magnet Project Director,
St. Luke's Episcopal Hospital, Houston, Texas

GINA LONG, DNSc, RN
Director of Nursing Research, Division of Nursing, Mayo Clinic College of Medicine,
Mayo Clinic Arizona, Mayo Clinic Hospital, Phoenix, Arizona

LISA ENGLISH LONG, MSN, RN, CNS
Director, Evidence-Based Practice, Center for Professional Excellence-Research and
Evidence-Based Practice, Cincinnati Children's Hospital Medical Center, Cincinnati, Ohio

JUNE MARSHALL, RN, MS, NEA-BC
Director, Center for Nurse Excellence, Medical City Hospital, Dallas, Texas

SUSAN McGEE, MSN, RN, CNP
Evidence-Based Practice Mentor, Center for Professional Excellence-Research and
Evidence-Based Practice, Cincinnati Children's Hospital Medical Center, Cincinnati, Ohio

PAMELA S. MILLER, RN, PhD(c), ACNP, CNS
Doctoral Candidate, University of California Los Angeles School of Nursing, Los Angeles,
California

MARILYN MOKRACEK, MSN, RN, CCRN, NE-BC
Nurse Manager, Neurosciences Services; and Chair, Best Practice Council, St. Luke's
Episcopal Hospital, Houston, Texas

CAROL MULVENON, MS, RN-BC, AOCN
Clinical Nurse Specialist, Pain Management, Palliative Care, Oncology, St. Joseph
Medical Center, Kansas City, Missouri

JULIE NEUMANN, MS, RN
Nursing Education Specialist and Instructor, Education and Professional Development
Division, Department of Nursing, Mayo Clinic Rochester, Rochester, Minnesota

MARIANNE OLSON, PhD, RN
Evidence-Based Practice Specialist, Nursing Research and Evidence-Based Practice
Division, Department of Nursing, Mayo Clinic Rochester, Rochester, Minnesota

JOE ONG, RN, BSN
Staff Nurse Evidence-Based Practice Fellow, Clinical Nurse III, Cardiothoracic Surgery Unit, Department of Nursing, Ronald Reagan University of California Los Angeles Medical Center, Los Angeles, California

DORRIN PATILLO, RN-B
Director of Staff Education, Education Department, Dorothea Dix Psychiatric Center, Bangor, Maine

TERI BRITT PIPE, PhD, RN
Director of Nursing Research; and Associate Professor, Division of Nursing, Mayo Clinic College of Medicine, Mayo Clinic Arizona, Mayo Clinic Hospital, Phoenix, Arizona

PATRICIA POTTER, PhD, RN, FAAN
Research Scientist, Siteman Cancer Center at Barnes-Jewish Hospital at Washington University Medical Center, St. Louis, Missouri

ELIZABETH PRATT, MSN, RN, ACNS-BC
Clinical Nurse Specialist, Barnes-Jewish Hospital, St. Louis, Missouri

GAIL REA, PhD, RN, CNE
Professor, Goldfarb School of Nursing at Barnes-Jewish College, St. Louis, Missouri

SARINA ROCHE, RNC, DNSc
Director of Nursing, Department of Nursing, Eastern Maine Community College, Bangor, Maine

CINDY SCHERB, PhD, RN
Clinical Nurse Researcher, Nursing Research Division, Department of Nursing, Mayo Clinic Rochester, Rochester, Minnesota

ALYCE A. SCHULTZ, PhD, RN, FAAN
President, EBP Concepts, Alyce A. Schultz & Associates, LLC, Chandler, Arizona

JEAN SMITH, RNC, BSN, MSN (c)
Manager of Clinical Operations, Neonatal Intensive Care Unit, Advocate Christ Medical Center/Hope Children's Hospital, Oak Lawn, Illinois

ANN E. SOSSONG, RN, PhD
Associate Professor/Undergraduate Coordinator, School of Nursing, University of Maine, Orono, Maine

ALANNA STETSON, RN, BSN, BC
Staff Developer, Education and Training Center, Eastern Maine Medical Center, Eastern Maine Healthcare, Brewer, Maine

J. WAYNE STREET, RN
Director, Trauma Center, Luther Midelfort, Eau Claire, Wisconsin

TANIA D. STROUT, RN, BSN, MS
Associate Director of Research, Maine Medical Center, Department of Emergency Medicine, Portland, Maine

PAULA THERIAULT, RN, MBA
Director of Education, Education Department, St. Joseph Hospital, Bangor, Maine

JANE A. TIMM, MS, RN
Informatics Nurse Specialist/NQF Scholars Project Manager, Nursing Research Division, Department of Nursing, Mayo Clinic Rochester, Rochester, Minnesota

SHARON TUCKER, PhD, RN
Nurse Administrator/Clinical Nurse Researcher, Nursing Research Division, Department of Nursing, Mayo Clinic Rochester, Rochester, Minnesota

WENDY TUZIK MICEK, PhD, RN
Director of Nursing Research and Professional Development, Advocate Christ Medical Center/Hope Children's Hospital, Oak Lawn, Illinois

DIANE TWEDELL, DNP, RN
Nurse Administrator, Education and Professional Development Division, Department of Nursing, Mayo Clinic Rochester, Rochester, Minnesota

LAURA WASZAK, RN
Nurse Clinician II, Neonatal Intensive Care Unit, Advocate Christ Medical Center/Hope Children's Hospital, Oak Lawn, Illinois

SUSAN MACE WEEKS, MS, RN, CNS-P/MH, LMFT, LCDC
Director, Center for Evidence-Based Practice and Research, Texas Christian University, Fort Worth, Texas

ROSANNA WELLING, RN, BSN, MBA
Clinical Operations Assistant, Neonatal Intensive Care Unit, Advocate Christ Medical Center/Hope Children's Hospital, Oak Lawn, Illinois

JENNIFER WILLIAMS, MSN, RN, ACNS-BC, CEN, CCRN
Clinical Nurse Specialist, Barnes-Jewish Hospital, St. Louis, Missouri

Contents

Preface   xv

Alyce A. Schultz

Unique Partnership and Collaborative Arrangements

**Evidence Equals Excellence: The Application of an Evidence-Based
Practice Model in an Academic Medical Center**   1

Karen Balakas, Patricia Potter, Elizabeth Pratt, Gail Rea,
and Jennifer Williams

> An evidence-based practice (EBP) program that is designed to develop
> mentors in both clinical and academic settings has the potential for trans-
> forming a health care organization. This article describes an innovative
> program, Evidence Equals Excellence, which consists of two components:
> a clinical practice component for health care clinicians and an academic
> program for baccalaureate and graduate nursing students. The develop-
> ment of EBP mentors creates a core group of clinicians who can assist fel-
> low staff members apply evidence at the bedside. An academic program
> prepares new graduates to partner easily with clinical mentors to support
> and initiate successful practice changes.

**A Collaborative Approach to Building the Capacity for Research and
Evidence-Based Practice in Community Hospitals**   11

Barbara B. Brewer, Melanie A. Brewer, and Alyce A. Schultz

> The use of best evidence to support nursing practice and the generation of
> new knowledge to use in practice are hallmarks of excellence. Nurses at
> the bedside, however, often lack the resources and knowledge necessary
> to change the traditional nursing culture to one in which the use of evi-
> dence is incorporated into daily care. This article describes the experience
> in two hospitals using a program designed to give nurses the skills needed
> to engage in evidence-based care.

**Development of an Evidence-Based Practice and Research Collaborative
Among Urban Hospitals**   27

Susan Mace Weeks, June Marshall, and Paulette Burns

> This article describes the development of an evidence-based practice and
> research collaborative among urban hospitals. The collaborative began as
> a mechanism to support the incorporation of evidence-based practice and
> research in the acute care practice setting. This article discusses the

development of the collaborative, as well as the challenges, success, and future goals from both the academic and practice perspectives.

Renewing the Spirit of Nursing: Embracing Evidence-Based Practice in a Rural State   33

Ann E. Sossong, Sue Cullen, Paula Theriault, Alanna Stetson, Barbara Higgins, Sarina Roche, Sue Ellis-Hermansen, and Dorrin Patillo

> A group of nursing leaders from several organizations in the central and northern regions of the state established the Maine Nursing Practice Consortium (MNPC). The MNPC has created educational opportunities through workshops that assist nurses with the development and implementation of evidence-based practice (EBP) in rural Maine. Through collaboration and consultation with EBP leaders, members have ignited a spirit of inquiry and gained the support of nurses from varied backgrounds to engage actively in EBP initiatives. This article briefly summarizes the process of establishing these collaborative partnerships, describes some of the outcomes from the workshops, and describes the organizational and individual commitment that was essential to the work.

Implementing a Health System–Wide Evidence-Based Practice Educational Program to Reach Nurses with Various Levels of Experience and Educational Preparation   43

Teri Britt Pipe, Jane A. Timm, Marcelline R. Harris, Doreen K. Frusti, Sharon Tucker, Jaqueline M. Attlesey-Pries, Katherine Brady-Schluttner, Julie Neumann, J. Wayne Street, Diane Twedell, Marianne Olson, Gina Long, and Cindy Scherb

> This article describes a system-wide evidence-based practice (EBP) educational initiative implemented with a geographically, educationally, and clinically diverse group of nurses with the intent of increasing their EBP skill set and efficacy as local change agents and leaders. The overall scope of the larger National Quality Forum Scholar Program is described, and then the focus is narrowed to describe the EBP components of the initiative with case examples and lessons learned.

Evidence-Based Practice at the Point-of-Care

Promotion of Safe Outcomes: Incorporating Evidence into Policies and Procedures   57

Lisa English Long, Karen Burkett, and Susan McGee

> This article describes the process of incorporating evidence into policies and procedures, resulting in the establishment of evidence as a basis for

safe practice. The process described includes use of the Rosswurm and Larrabee model for change to evidence-based practice. The model guided the work of evidence-based practice mentors in developing a template, system, and educational plan for dissemination of evidence-based policies and procedures into patient care.

Staff Nurses Creating Safe Passage with Evidence-Based Practice   71

Dora Bradley and John F. Dixon

Patient safety is one of the most critical issues for health care today. The escalating need to decrease preventable complications serves as a significant catalyst to identify and use evidence-based practice (EBP) at the bedside. Decreasing preventable complications requires a synergistic relationship between the nurses at the bedside and nursing leadership. This article presents an overview of the concepts and the specific structures and processes used at Baylor Health Care System to increase the use of EBP and improve patient safety.

A Nursing Quality Program Driven by Evidence-Based Practice   83

Jacqueline J. Anderson, Marilyn Mokracek, and Cheryl N. Lindy

St. Luke's Episcopal Hospital in Houston established a best-practice council as a strategy to link nursing quality to evidence-based practice. Replacing a system based on reporting quality control and compliance, this Best Practice Council formed interdisciplinary teams, charged them each with a quality issue, and directed them to change practice as needed under the guidance of the St. Luke's Episcopal Hospital Evidence Based Practice Model. This article reviews the activities of the Best Practice Council and the projects of teams assigned to study best practice in (1) preventing bloodstream infection (related to central lines), (2) preventing patient falls, (3) assessing and preventing pressure ulcers, and (4) ensuring good hand-off communication.

Development and Implementation of an Inductive Model for Evidence-Based Practice: A Grassroots Approach for Building Evidence-Based Practice Capacity in Staff Nurses   93

Tania D. Strout, Kelly Lancaster, and Alyce A. Schultz

Evidence-based practice (EBP) is an essential component of the development of nursing science and has importance for today's clinical nurses. It benefits patients, organizations, and the nursing discipline, as well as having personal and professional benefits for individual clinicians. As interest in EBP has grown, so has the need for educational programs designed to develop the scholarly skills of the nursing workforce. The Clinical Scholar Model is one grassroots approach to developing a cadre of clinical nurses who have the EBP and research skills necessary in today's demanding health care delivery environments.

Effect of a Preoperative Instructional Digital Video Disc on Patient Knowledge and Preparedness for Engaging in Postoperative Care Activities   103

Joe Ong, Pamela S. Miller, Renee Appleby, Rebecca Allegretto, and Anna Gawlinski

This project determined the effects of developing and implementing a preoperative instructional digital video disc (DVD) on patients' level of knowledge, preparedness, and perceived ability to participate in postoperative care activities. Content areas that were incorporated into the preoperative instructional DVD included: pain management, surgical drainage, vital signs, incentive spirometry, cough and deep breathe, chest physiotherapy, anti-embolism stockings/sequential compression device, ambulation, diet/bowel activity/urine output, and discharge. A system was created to ensure that patients consistently received the preoperative instructional DVD prior to surgery. The instructional media product was found to be effective in increasing pre-operative knowledge and preparedness of patients and their families. Nurses reported higher levels of knowledge and engagement among patients and their families related to postoperative activities.

The Clinical Scholar Model: Evidence-Based Practice at the Bedside   117

Cynthia Honess, Paulette Gallant, and Kathleen Keane

The Clinical Scholar Model serves as an effective framework for investigating and implementing evidence-based practice (EBP) changes by direct care providers. The model guides one in identifying problems and issues, key stakeholders, and the need for practice changes. It provides a framework to critique and synthesize the external and internal evidence. Three EBP projects conducted at a large tertiary care facility in northern New England illustrate the process of using the Clinical Scholar Model.

Using Evidence to Improve Care for the Vulnerable Neonatal Population   131

Cheryl A. Lefaiver, Phyllis Lawlor-Klean, Rosanna Welling, Jean Smith, Laura Waszak, and Wendy Tuzik Micek

The facilitation of evidence-based practice (EBP) in the clinical setting is important to ensure patients receive the best care possible. This article highlights changes in open visitation and feeding readiness practices that occurred in a Magnet-designated facility neonatal ICU. The examples demonstrate ways to bring evidence to the bedside within an environment that supports EBP at all levels of nursing leadership.

From the Bedside to the Boardroom: Resuscitating the Use of Nursing Research   **145**

Carol Mulvenon and M. Kathleen Brewer

> This article describes the process used by a multi-institutional organization to engage nurses in using and conducting nursing research using the Clinical Scholar Model. The challenges faced on the journey to engage nurses in questioning their practice and searching for answers are highlighted. Key resources necessary for a successful outcome are identified.

Index   **153**

FORTHCOMING ISSUES

June 2009
Long-Term Care
Linda Dumas, PhD, RN, ANP,
Guest Editor

September 2009
**Legal and Ethical Issues: To Know,
To Reason, To Act**
Dana Bjarnason, RN, MA, CNA, PhD
and Michele A. Carter, PhD, RN,
Guest Editors

December 2009
Women's Health
Ellen Olshansky, DNSc, RNC, FAAN,
Guest Editor

RECENT ISSUES

December 2008
**Technology: The Interface to Nursing
Educational Informatics**
Elizabeth E. Weiner, PhD, RN-BC, FAAN,
Guest Editor

September 2008
Vulnerable Populations
Marcia Stanhope, RN, DSN, FAAN,
Lisa M. Turner, MSN, APRN, BC,
and Peggy Riley, RN, MSN,
Guest Editors

June 2008
Oncology Nursing: Past, Present, and Future
Marilyn Frank-Stromborg, MS, EdD, JD, FAAN,
and Judith Johnson, PhD, RN, FAAN,
Guest Editors

Preface

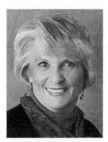

Alyce A. Schultz, RN, PhD, FAAN
Guest Editor

Over 150 years ago, Florence Nightingale taught us that one of the most important practical lessons we can give student nurses is to always observe: teaching them what to observe; how to observe; and which symptoms are important for indicating improvement, decline, or neglect. She further instructed that as nurses, we should not spend our time collecting voluminous amounts of data that we do not use to improve the care we provide to our patients and that handwashing prevents the spread of infection.[1] How can we still be struggling with using our keen observation skills to improve care, collecting data that we do not use and spending millions of dollars attempting to sustain the evidence-based practice of handwashing?

If you have ever attempted to execute practice changes in your setting, particularly if the changes required support from multiple disciplines and administration, you know how complicated and challenging implementing evidence-based practice can be. Critique and synthesis of a body of research literature and changes in practice that are dramatic changes from the traditional way of care further challenge change efforts. In an effort to implement short-term solutions, quick fixes are put into practice, with practices steeped in tradition or "the way we have always done things." Senge and colleagues[2] directed us to pay more attention to long-term solutions with our practice issues, using programs that promote a sustainable change, creating and sustaining a learning environment in which point-of-care providers have the resources and knowledge necessary to improve patient outcomes through the use of best evidence. Building the capacity for evidence-based practice at the point-of-care provides a long-term solution to changing patterns of thinking and providing evidence-based care.

Medicine is often credited with the initiation of evidence-based practice; yet, in the mid- to late 1970s, researchers at Western Institute of Collegiate Education in Nursing (WICHEN) studied barriers to the use of research in nursing practice, the same barriers we find today. The Conduct and Utilization of Research in Nursing project examined the research evidence supporting or changing the care we were providing and published 10 practices that had sufficient scientific evidence. The definition for using research in practice at that point in time was research utilization. Concurrently, Dr. Archie Cochrane admonished his fellow physicians for their lack of research utilization in guiding their practice decisions. In the 1990s, Sackett and colleagues expanded thinking for incorporating more sources of evidence than just research findings in making clinical decisions regarding care. The Institute of Medicine's landmark reports *To Err Is Human* and *Crossing the Quality Chasm: A New Health System for the 21st Century* brought a new awareness to the important decision-making issues of quality and safety facing patients and clinicians alike in our complex health care system.[3] Building on the 3 decades of work in nursing and medicine, the thrust from regulatory and credentialing agencies, and the nationwide efforts to build centers of nursing excellence supported by the Magnet Recognition Program from the American Nurses Credentialing Center, evidence-based health care has become the mantra for managing and changing our practice in the twenty-first century.

Use of the best evidence to support nursing practice and the generation of new knowledge to use in practice are the hallmarks of excellence across the nation and the globe. Yet, studies continue to find that nurses at the bedside are limited in the resources and knowledge necessary to change the traditional nursing culture to one in which the use of evidence is incorporated into daily care.[4] In the hectic world of today's nurse, finding the time to explore clinical and administrative questions systematically often takes a back seat to ever increasing demands of patient care and the work environment. This issue provides a wide array of examples representing the current thinking in and the efforts for establishing evidence-based health care, with continual improvement of patient outcomes.

The issue is organized around two themes, although, as you are likely to note in your reading, there is overlap between and among the articles. The first theme offers a multiplicity of unique partnerships and collaborative efforts used to facilitate evidence-based practice within educational and service settings. The articles within this section describe a unique program within a large academic medical center that addresses nursing education and nursing practice, one example of various joint agreements between an academic institution and clinical settings with multiple benefits, two collaborative strategies among multiple academic centers and multiple health care facilities (one in an urban setting and one in a rural setting), and, finally, a unique Web-based program used by a large multisite health care system to meet the needs of its staff in multiple geographic sites.

The second theme provides a rich collection of point-of-care exemplars. These exemplars include a template for planning and implementing strategies for evidence-based policies and procedures and a synergistic professional practice model that incorporates evidence-based practice and a nursing quality model that drives evidence-based care. Examples of the background on clinical questions, the search and synthesis of the evidence, and improvements in patient outcomes provide evidence-based ideas for use in other settings or opportunities for replication projects addressing important, relevant, common practice issues in a diversity of patient populations. This section concludes with a reflective article on challenges and opportunities in implementing the conduct of research and the use of evidence throughout a nursing department in a health care system.

Several models and frameworks for promoting and sustaining evidence-based practice are available for guidance on your journey toward improvement in patient care based on the best evidence. The articles in this section provide you with the references for a diverse group of models that can be used and further tested by individuals and small groups in addition to organizational models that can facilitate assessing and changing the larger work environment. Clearly, one model does not fit all organizations and all work settings or units. Selection of a model based on your workforce mix and resources is an important initial step in creating and sustaining a work environment in which the spirit of inquiry thrives and the best available evidence is incorporated into daily decisions for health care.

Almost 30 years ago, at a conference sponsored by the WICHEN entitled "Promoting Nursing Research as a Staff Nursing Function," Dr. Janelle Krueger declared that if research were ever to be valued and used, staff nurses must know how to read and conduct research studies because they are the individuals who know the important clinical questions. Dr. Krueger went on to say there would never be enough doctorally prepared nurses at the bedside to ask the questions. My own journey into creating an environment in which direct care providers would have the knowledge and support needed to conduct their own research and utilize these scientific findings, along with their expert knowledge, was sparked by her words. It is indeed an honor to bring you an issue packed with the knowledge transfer work of nurse educators, administrators, advanced practice nurses, and bedside staff.

It has been a privilege to serve as the guest editor of this timely issue on evidence-based practice. Building the capacity for evidence-based practice at the point of care provides a long-term solution to changing patterns of thinking through promotion of the use of evidence and generation of new knowledge. Sustaining a learning environment in which point-of-care providers have the resources and knowledge necessary to improve patient outcomes through the use of best evidence requires unique partnerships with academic programs and within and among health care systems. Nursing leadership must be knowledgeable and support the resources needed in the future work environment. I hope that this issue provides you with many ideas for the future.

Alyce A. Schultz, RN, PhD, FAAN
EBP Concepts
Alyce A. Schultz & Associates, LLC
5747 West Drake Court
Chandler, AZ 85226

E-mail address:
alyceaschultz@gmail.com

REFERENCES

1. Nightingale F. Notes on nursing: what it is, and what it is not. New York: D. Appleton and Company; 1898. Available at: http://www.gutenberg.org/etext/12439. Accessed July 24, 2008.
2. Senge P, Kleiner A, Roberts C, et al. The dance of change: the challenges of sustaining momentum in learning organizations. New York: Doubleday; 1999.
3. Committee on the Quality of Health Care in America, Institute of Medicine. Crossing the quality chasm: a new health system for the 21st century. Washington, DC: National Academies Press; 2001.
4. Pravikoff DS, Tanner AB, Pierce ST. Readiness of US nurses for evidence-based practice. Am J Nurs 2005;105:40–51.

Evidence Equals Excellence: The Application of an Evidence-Based Practice Model in an Academic Medical Center

Karen Balakas, PhD, RN, CNE[a], Patricia Potter, PhD, RN, FAAN[b],*,
Elizabeth Pratt, MSN, RN, ACNS-BC[c], Gail Rea, PhD, RN, CNE[a],
Jennifer Williams, MSN, RN, ACNS-BC, CEN, CCRN[c]

KEYWORDS

- Clinical • Education • Evidence-based practice • Mentoring
- Practice change

Within today's health care environment, there are numerous initiatives for health care organizations to adopt evidence-based practice (EBP) as a framework for the ongoing development and improvement of clinical practice. EBP is a problem-solving approach to clinical practice that integrates the conscientious use of best evidence in combination with a clinician's expertise and patient preferences and values in making decisions about patient care.[1,2] Patient safety and economic initiatives have triggered efforts at adopting EBP models within health care organizations to reduce patient injury, control costs, and improve the quality of patient care. Accrediting agencies such as The Joint Commission and credentialing programs such as the Magnet Recognition Program have incorporated research and EBP as underlying themes necessary for organizations to ensure health care excellence. In two quality-related reports, the Institute of Medicine[3] emphasized the importance of applying EBP to ensure the use of best practices and improve the education of health care professionals.[4]

[a] Goldfarb School of Nursing at Barnes-Jewish College, Mailstop 9060697, 4483 Duncan Avenue, St. Louis, MO 63110, USA
[b] Siteman Cancer Center at Barnes-Jewish Hospital at Washington University School of Medicine, Box 8100, 660 S. Euclid, St. Louis, MO 63110, USA
[c] Barnes-Jewish Hospital, Mailstop 9059360, 1 Barnes-Jewish Hospital Plaza, St. Louis, MO 63110, USA
* Corresponding author.
E-mail address: pap1212@bjc.org (P. Potter).

Nurs Clin N Am 44 (2009) 1–10
doi:10.1016/j.cnur.2008.10.001
0029-6465/08/$ – see front matter © 2009 Elsevier Inc. All rights reserved.

EVIDENCE-BASED PRACTICE IN AN ACADEMIC SETTING

In a large academic medical center, various levels of bureaucracy and associated decision processes often make change difficult. To implement an EBP program with promise of permanence, EBP must become part of the cultural fabric of an organization. An EBP program that is designed to develop mentors in both clinical and academic settings has the potential for transforming a health care organization. The EBP program at Barnes-Jewish Hospital at Washington University Medical Center and the Goldfarb School of Nursing at Barnes-Jewish College is innovative. The program, Evidence Equals Excellence (EEE), focuses on the education and mentoring of clinicians and nursing students to foster a level of clinical inquiry needed to make EBP a philosophy of clinical practice.

Barnes-Jewish Hospital at Washington University Medical Center is an academic teaching hospital licensed for 1200 beds. The hospital enjoys a long relationship with the Goldfarb School of Nursing at Barnes-Jewish College. The hospital also has a long-standing involvement in nursing research, and the school of nursing faculty routinely has partnered with the hospital in research and educational programs. In the fall of 2005, an EBP team of clinicians, faculty, and a nursing research scientist developed EEE, a unique EBP program. The program has two components: a clinical practice component for health care clinicians and an academic program for baccalaureate and graduate nursing students. The EBP model used in the EEE program is adapted from the Advancing Research and Clinical Practice through Close Collaboration model created by Melnyk and Fineout-Overholt[2,5] at Arizona State University. The goal of the EEE program is to develop evidence-based practice mentors and clinicians who are equipped to lead the effort in using evidence to improve nursing practice.

DEVELOPING THE EVIDENCE EQUALS EXCELLENCE PROGRAM

The impetus for the EEE program began when team members attended the Arizona State University's EBP mentorship program, a 5-day immersion program designed to prepare organizational leaders and mentors in changing organizational cultures through the promotion, implementation, and sustainability of EBP. The strength of the Arizona State model for EBP lies in its adaptability to any health care organizational structure. It does not require a major change in an organization's infrastructure.

At Barnes-Jewish Hospital, a shared governance model is in place with unit practice committees on each nursing unit (many are multidisciplinary) and a central practice committee that meets monthly. The hospital also has a large presence of advanced practice nurses who, when trained on EBP principles, provide a solid staff resource for making practice changes. With a sound infrastructure in place, the EEE program prepares mentors who then can assist staff in making practice changes relatively quickly.

Members of the EEE team quickly became champions of EBP principles, an important characteristic needed to guide the EBP process for an organization.[6] The team had a vision: to develop an EBP program for the hospital and school that can generate clinical EBP mentors who champion practice changes at the nursing unit level. From the beginning, the EEE team was committed to making its work both fun and challenging. Among the five members were clinicians, educators, previous managers and directors of nursing, and researchers. The variety of talent contributed to lively planning meetings and a continuous source of ideas necessary to make the program relevant and current. The EEE program is always changing because of the new ideas team members offer for program, course, and individual mentor development.

The Clinical Program

The clinical practice component consists of a 2-day multidisciplinary seminar for mentors, a semiannual refresher program for mentors, and a 4-hour class (the Champions Class) for clinicians. The team members are the faculty for the program and a library scientist from Washington University.

Two-day seminar

The 2-day seminar is structured along the six-step model from the Arizona State University program (**Box 1**). An introduction to EBP is followed by individual lectures and group work on each of the six steps (**Box 2**). The seminar is highly participative. Before the seminar, participants are asked to submit clinical questions regarding their area of interest so that faculty can integrate questions relevant to participants in the appropriate presentations. For example, participants spend 2 hours learning how to develop clinical questions, using a population of interest/intervention of interest/comparative intervention/outcome (PICO) format. Questions framed in a PICO format improve success in obtaining relevant articles during a literature search. During the seminar participants have the opportunity to rephrase their own questions as well as those of their colleagues. The aim of this exercise is to help participants develop questions that will lead to EBP projects on their work units.

A particularly popular presentation in the seminar is "Searching the Literature." A library scientist uses participant questions to demonstrate literature searches. Using popular databases such as PubMed, MEDLINE, the Cumulative Index to Nursing and Allied Health Literature (CINAHL), and the Cochrane Library, participants learn advanced search techniques that prepare them to search the literature for the best scientific evidence. In everyday clinical practice, it is imperative for an EBP mentor to be able to retrieve a few relevant articles that pertain to a clinical question or problem. The advanced search techniques include approaches in using search limits and search filters and tips on navigating different databases.

The seminar also includes presentations on research methods and on critiquing the evidence that give participants the opportunity, through group work, to recognize different study designs in the literature and how to review journal articles. The group process expedites the review, gives the participants experience in working within a group to review articles, and helps participants realize that most clinicians need help in appraising research articles. Participants receive copies of critical appraisal guidelines (developed by Melnyk and Fineout-Overholt) for the different types of research (eg, randomized, controlled trials or quasi-experimental or qualitative studies).

In the presentation on "How to Make Evidence Work at the Bedside," a faculty member, who is one of the clinical specialists, shares stories about actual EBP

Box 1
The six steps of evidence-based practice

1. Ask a burning clinical question
2. Collect the best evidence
3. Review the evidence critically
4. Integrate the evidence
5. Evaluate outcomes
6. Communicate results

| Box 2 |
| Outline for the Evidence Equals Excellence seminar |
| *Day 1* |
| Evidence-based practice: the path to excellence |
| Developing PICO questions |
| Research designs |
| Searching the literature for evidence |
| Laboratory practice: searching evidence |
| *Day 2* |
| Appraisal of the evidence |
| Being a change agent for EBP |
| Panel of EBP mentors |
| Outcomes measurement |
| Making EBP work at the bedside |

programs implemented by her unit mentors. The seminar also includes a panel presentation by previous mentors, who discuss ongoing projects and share stories of their experiences in implementing EBP. These two presentations are very popular because they allow the participants to hear stories from past mentors about actual EBP projects, the challenges and barriers to implementation, and the approaches that result in successful implementation.

Refresher program

To date more than 100 nurses, social workers, respiratory therapists, and radiology technologists have attended the EEE seminars. A series of semiannual refresher programs keeps the mentors informed about current EBP activities and opportunities. These programs are valuable in giving mentors time to discuss strategies for work-unit implementation. Mentors discuss ongoing projects, the approaches used to involve staff, and project outcomes. Frequently mentors share ideas that have relevant applications for other units attempting similar projects. For example, several units have introduced hourly nurse rounds as an EBP fall-prevention project. The approaches for improving staff compliance with a rounding protocol on one unit can be useful for staff on other units as well.

The champions class

An abbreviated version of the EEE seminar was designed to educate bedside clinicians who are unable to commit to a mentoring role. After identifying the critical components from the 2-day EEE seminar, the two clinical nurse specialists on the EEE team coordinated the Champions Class. They encourage proficient staff from all disciplines to attend. Shift changes dictate the scheduling of classes, and attendees request specific dates amenable to staffing schedules. The class commences with an overview of EBP, emphasizing the knowledge explosion in nursing and the initiatives leading to a mandate of EBP. The class highlights the basics of EBP and prepares staff to become competent in EBP language, to partner with mentors, and to support best-practice implementation.

The EEE team recognizes the need for change agents to create a culture of EBP. Duck's Change Curve Model shows that group change requires individual change, and the greater the number of individuals involved, the more difficult effecting change will be.[7] Thus, hospital mentors require multiple champions to support their belief in the value of applying EBP and their initiatives in doing so.

Staff members are eager to implement best practices but may be overwhelmed by the thought of conducting a literature search and appraising the studies. Changing the hospital's culture to one that envelops EBP requires support and enthusiasm from clinicians at all levels. The EEE team asks mentors who graduate from the seminar to recruit expert staff members from their work units to attend the 3-hour Champions Class. Through the Champions Class, the program prepares a considerable number of caregivers who learn to understand the significance of searching for and using best evidence in practice. Ploeg and colleagues[8] highlighted 10 published studies that focused on facilitators and barriers to implementing best practice. The authors noted that one of the most common themes was the presence of change champions. The involvement of bedside clinicians is critical to change the environment to one that embraces clinical inquiry or the questioning and evaluating of best practices.

The Champions Class adapts content for relevance to the participants' clinical backgrounds, and the clinical nurse specialists encourage interactive discussion of traditional but not necessarily evidence-based practices that are ingrained in the hospital. As in the mentor seminar, the participants submit clinical questions before the class. The faculty discusses how to establish a culture of clinical inquiry by asking relevant clinical questions. The faculty then assists the participants in formulating their questions using the PICO format. Staff with little research experience report that they have difficulty searching the literature. Structuring their questions in the PICO format helps the participants outline their clinical question clearly and simplifies the search. The participants are most engaged when the discussion leads to the identification of practice issues and how they can use EBP to improve clinical outcomes.

Conducting the Champions Class has led the faculty to recognize that nurses are seeking a guide that will help them make decisions that are accurate and timely to apply evidence in the practice setting.[9] The class ends with an emphasis on working with the EBP mentors and resources available in the hospital. The clinical nurse specialists encourage participants to access the EBP intranet Web site, which provides staff with the steps of EBP, links to search engines, and EBP mentors and their ongoing projects.

Successful implementation of an EBP practice culture relies heavily on knowledge and belief in the value of EBP. More than 50 staff members representing the disciplines of nursing, respiratory therapy, and social work have attended the Champions Class to date. These EBP advocates have been involved in numerous projects throughout the hospital. Champions participate in journal clubs and quality improvement initiatives identified through their unit practice committees. Examples of projects by mentors and champions include the implementation of bedside reporting, a new tube-feeding protocol, fall-prevention rounds, and family presence during resuscitation efforts. As more disciplines participate in the class, participants are able to share their applications of best practice and encourage others to employ these changes in their work areas. Most importantly, participants learn the EBP language and promote discussion of why they choose specific practices. Participants become engaged in applying research and are able to communicate effectively with other disciplines, notably physicians. An educated staff increases scholarly discussions and elevates professionalism among the disciplines.

The Academic Program

During the past decade there has been a paradigm shift in teaching from a traditional nursing curriculum to one that supports and prepares nurses to practice in an evidence-based environment.[10–12] Following the Institute of Medicine's Quality Chasm series,[3] the Health Professions Educational Summit[13] identified five core competencies that all educators need to address within a curriculum:

Providing patient-centered care
Working in interdisciplinary teams
Employing EBP
Applying quality improvement
Using informatics

Many schools have responded to this mandate and incorporated EBP into their programs. It is far easier, however, to talk about the need to teach EBP than it is actually to accomplish the task.

Across the country, research courses have been revised to address the steps of EBP,[14–16] and additional courses have been developed to support further student development in the use of EBP.[15,17,18] Informatics courses are invaluable in helping students learn to search the literature effectively and in introducing databases such as The Cochrane Library (which contains four databases), CINAHL, MEDLINE, and PubMed. Clinical decision making relies on the ability to access and appraise research results; thus, education in how to find the best available evidence is critical for EBP. Some research courses teach students how to construct an evidence-based analysis and may incorporate a journal club to help teach appraisal skills.[10,18] Courses with a clinical component frequently incorporate assignments that include creating an answerable PICO question, requiring students to search the literature to find an answer, and communicating their findings.[15]

In the fall of 2005, the hospital and college collaborated in sponsoring a conference on EBP and invited Drs. Melnyk and Fineout-Overholt from Arizona State University. The hospital recently had achieved Magnet status and was working with the college to promote baccalaureate education among the nursing staff. As part of that initiative, the hospital was preparing to fund the education of 200 nurses. Following the conference, a special workshop was facilitated by the speakers for the Goldfarb School of Nursing faculty to learn how to incorporate EBP into a curriculum. The faculty on the EEE team elected to help lead the effort to revise the Registered Nurse/Bachelor of Science in Nursing (RN-BSN) curriculum to incorporate EBP for a new cohort of nurses from the hospital who would be taking the program in an online format.

The faculty and clinicians on the EEE team collaborated to explore ways to engage RN-BSN graduates in EBP upon completion of their academic program. Because the graduates would be learning the essential skills necessary for EBP, changes would have to be made in the hospital environment so the graduates could have the opportunity to apply their knowledge and continue to practice evidence-based nursing. This partnership of educators and clinicians, through the EEE program, has promoted change within the hospital with the development of EBP mentors and champions. The ultimate goal of the academic program is to partner new graduates with unit-based EBP mentors to support and initiate successful practice changes.

Initially, EBP was incorporated fully into the school's online RN-BSN curriculum. Although faculty had brought the curriculum outline back from the immersion workshop at Arizona State University, the faculty as a whole worked to develop each of the courses. Faculty divided into teams and applied the concepts learned in previous workshops with the guidance of faculty mentors. As students begin the program, they are introduced to change theory and models for EBP. Assignments within the beginning courses focus on the construction of PICO questions and how to search the literature effectively. The nursing research course is positioned early in the curriculum to emphasize the steps of EBP and to help students learn how to appraise studies critically. In the course, students develop a PICO question and then construct an evidence-based analysis to arrive at an answer. In subsequent nursing courses, students are challenged to begin projects within their work setting to illustrate EBP. For example, students have created PICO question boxes on their units, developed posters to illustrate the steps of EBP, and participated in EBP projects with mentors who attended the EEE seminar.

The incorporation of EBP into the online curriculum generated positive feedback from students and faculty. As a result, each of the courses within the remaining baccalaureate programs has been redesigned with a new description, course outcomes, and assignments that support the development of EBP. Faculty members strive to create at least one assignment within each course that furthers understanding and application of EBP. Students develop PICO questions in each of the clinical courses and share the evidence they find to answer their questions with peers and the nursing staff on their practicum unit. During one of the semesters, students worked with managers from the community outreach department of a local pediatric hospital to determine whether the programs being offered in the community were evidence based. Students shared their findings with the hospital management and were able to see the impact of their analysis as changes were proposed for the programs.

The graduate program also was revised to emphasize EBP and the new role expectations for advanced-practice nurses. Students continue to develop PICO questions as they complete clinical hours and now are expected to use their findings to guide decision making at point of care. Students have revised clinical protocols, such as the guideline now used at a National Cancer Institute–designated cancer center for central venous catheter dressing changes in neutropenic patients. Some of the evidence-based analyses that students have completed have led to research studies on their units. For example, students were interested in the use of chewing gum to promote gastrointestinal motility in postoperative colorectal patients. They concluded that the evidence was not strong enough to support a practice change and now are conducting a study to confirm their findings.

Communicating the results is an important component of EBP and is part of the academic programs. Students have developed posters and papers that have been presented at local and statewide research conferences. Developing a poster and an abstract with an evidence-based analysis is an assignment in the graduate research course. The capstone project for the graduate program reflects the application of EBP and supports the student's role as an EBP mentor and change-agent upon graduation.

A CASE STUDY: MAKING EVIDENCE-BASED PRACTICE WORK AT THE BEDSIDE

EBP can be infused into the work culture of a hospital department in multiple ways. Strategies for implementation include developing policy and procedures, creating work teams focused on nursing interventions, integrating EBP concepts into employee performance expectations, and purposeful recruiting of new employees who are familiar with EBP concepts. Within the emergency department (ED), all these approaches have been embraced and used to enhance the nurse's role as an active and informed partner in patient care.

The policies and procedures in the ED are developed and reviewed annually for currency and relevance. As part of this process the procedure and references are verified using the PICO method to assure that all changes and updates are evidence based. An example of this practice involved the revision of the triage policy to include an alcohol screening by the nursing staff. Recent guidelines[19,20] demonstrated the value of including a brief alcohol consumption screen by the nurse and pairing it with a short intervention. This screen was added to the triage policy along with a list of resources for individuals who may be at risk for binge drinking or alcoholism. The nurse provides the list of resources to the patient upon completing the screen. The next step in this process will be the full implementation of the brief intervention by the nurse when a patient has a positive screening. A rewarding finding from this practice implementation has been seeing patients who screened positively for at-risk alcohol consumption and who were admitted later asking for assistance and resources. The initial screening seems to stimulate the conversation about alcohol use and to encourage at-risk individuals to consider assistance.

The value in demonstrating that nursing polices and practices are evidence based has created a culture in the department in which staff members routinely seek out the evidence that supports treatment decisions. All members of the treatment team are encouraged to inquire about the evidence supporting a practice, especially when nurses and physicians are discussing the plan of care. In addition, the physician residency program supports and encourages the use of EBP. The physicians host a monthly EBP journal club that all physicians and ED nursing staff are welcome to attend. The topics reflect ongoing developments in clinical practice, and the forum is used to explore new treatment approaches the department is considering adopting. This support has led to a practice environment that encourages open discussion and values the input from all team members.

The clinical nurse specialist in the ED, who is an EEE faculty member, developed a cadre of staff nurses in both formal and informal leadership roles as EBP mentors. Ten direct-care nursing staff members have attended the EEE seminar in the past 2 years. As this group formed, they began to develop unit-specific patient care questions and, as a team, used the tools they had acquired at the workshop. The team began by identifying a single practice question: what is the evidence to support a practice change for supported family presence during medical resuscitation? The group reviewed the current literature and developed a consensus document in support of the practice. The team determined that family presence should be implemented in the ED and then sought administrative support. Providing the nursing and physician leadership with an evidence-based position statement facilitated the formal implementation of the program. The ED EBP team then identified the opportunity to develop the project into a formal research study regarding the staff beliefs about the practice of family presence. After seeking Human Studies Committee approval, the team distributed the pre-implementation survey and used the results to develop and expand the education and training plan. A post-implementation survey was distributed 6 months after the initial survey to evaluate whether changes had occurred in the department. Statistically significant improvement ($P < .05$) in staff members' willingness to have family present at the bedside during resuscitation or invasive procedures was achieved.

The changes regarding family presence are an excellent example of the impact of EBP in patient care. The group continues to grow and address other concerns in the department including skin care, the effective use of capnography, and the use of noninvasive technology to assess tissue oxygenation and stroke volume. The team communicates their findings to the department via posters, monthly newsletters, e-mail, and through the unit practice committee.

The ED EBP team members participate actively on specific disease process–focused committees within the department. As members of those core clinical practice treatment teams, they are able to represent the larger nursing staff and can address issues brought forward using an EBP approach. Examples of clinical practice teams that benefit from this input are the acute stroke tissue plasminogen activator reperfusion team, acute myocardial treatment team, pneumonia treatment team, and sepsis treatment team. Focusing the teams on an EBP framework has streamlined and standardized care among the large numbers of nursing and physician staff, resulting in positive patient outcomes that have been sustained over time.

Approaching recruitment and retention through an EBP model also has led to changes. Potential candidates for the ED are assessed to determine their level of familiarity with EBP concepts and how these concepts are related strategically to their position in the department. One successful example of this philosophy was the hire of a new graduate nurse who had attended the college's RN-BSN program that empha- sized EBP. He had used EBP throughout his academic program to identify clinical patient care issues and address the appropriate nursing interventions with evidence support. Once graduated, he actively sought a department that would embrace excel- lent clinical nursing practice and incorporate evidence into its care structure. Conse- quently, he chose the ED. During his first year as a nurse in the ED, he became involved in the use of evidence-based protocols for the management of the patients who had suffered an acute myocardial infarction and of septic patients. He was able to identify multiple opportunities to develop and implement EBP as they relate to fall prevention in the ED and is redesigning the current standards. He will attend the EEE mentorship workshop in the future to develop further his literature searching strategies and to focus his clinical practice questions.

Actively engaging the staff in the practice of EBP has implications for retention.[21,22] As part of the performance appraisal process, employees in the ED receive feedback on their individual performance in relation to the core clinical practice measures. Meet- ing those measures is a role expectation in the unit. The nurses report that they feel a sense of ownership of the EBP process and subsequent practice changes. Promot- ing a sense of autonomy has decreased the staff turnover and created a positive environment.

SUMMARY

The application of EBP within a large, academic medical center requires an infrastruc- ture to support practice change as well as the development of clinicians and students who become adept at using EBP principles. The partnering of clinicians and academic faculty in developing an EBP program brings together multiple talents and perspec- tives to create a program that is innovative, dynamic, and diverse. The EEE program has been successful in preparing clinicians to apply EBP principles and in creating an environment where they can successfully make changes to improve practice, quality of care, and patient and staff satisfaction.

ACKNOWLEDGMENT

The authors acknowledge the support of JoAnn O'Neill, RN, in the review of this article.

REFERENCES

1. Sackett DL, Straus SE, Richardson WS, et al. Evidence-based medicine: how to practice and teach EBM. London: Churchill Livingstone; 2000.
2. Melnyk BM, Fineout-Overholt E. Making the case for evidence-based practice. In: Melnyk BM, Fineout-Overholt E, editors. Evidence-based practice in nursing &

healthcare: a guide to best practice. Philadelphia: Lippincott, Williams & Wilkins; 2005. p. 3–24.

3. Institute of Medicine. Crossing the quality chasm: a new health system for the 21st century. Washington, DC: National Academy Press; 2001.
4. Greiner AA, Knebel E, editors. Health professions education: a bridge to quality. Washington, DC: National Academy Press; 2003.
5. Melnyk BM, Fineout-Overholt E. Consumer preferences and values as an integral key to evidence-based practice. Nurs Adm Q 2006;30(2):123–7.
6. Fineout-Overholt E, Levin RF, Melnyk BM. Strategies for advancing evidence-based practice in clinical settings. J N Y State Nurses Assoc 2005;35(2):28–32.
7. Duck JD. The change monster: the human forces that fuel or foil corporate transformation and change. New York: Crown Business; 2001.
8. Ploeg J, Davies B, Edwards N, et al. Factors influencing best-practice guideline implementation: lessons learned from administrators, nursing staff, and project leaders. Worldviews Evid Based Nurs 2007;4(4):210–9.
9. Newhouse R, Dearholt S, Poe S, et al. Evidence-based practice: a practical approach to implementation. J Nurs Adm 2005;35(1):35–40.
10. Burke L, Schlenk E, Sereika S, et al. Developing research competence to support evidence-based practice. J Prof Nurs 2005;21(6):358–63.
11. Callister L, Matsumura G, Lookinland S, et al. Inquiry in baccalaureate nursing education: fostering evidence-based practice. J Nurs Educ 2005;44(2):59–64.
12. Fineout-Overholt E, Johnson L. Teaching EBP: a challenge for educators in the 21st century. Worldviews Evid Based Nurs 2005;2(1):37–9.
13. Committee on the Health Professions Education Summit. Health professions education: a bridge to quality. Washington, DC: The National Academies Press; 2003. Available at: http://books.nap.edu/openbook.php?record_id=10681&;page=1. Accessed April 7, 2008.
14. Ciliska D. Educating for evidence-based practice. J Prof Nurs 2005;21(6):345–50.
15. Brancato V. An innovative clinical practicum to teach evidence-based practice. Nurse Educ 2006;31(5):195–9.
16. Ferguson L, Day R. Evidence-based nursing education: myth or reality? J Nurs Educ 2005;44(3):107–15.
17. Courey T, Benson-Soros J, Deemer K. The missing link: information literacy and evidence-based practice as a new challenge for nurse educators. Nurs Educ Perspect 2006;27(6):320–3.
18. Killeen M, Barnfather J. A successful teaching strategy for applying evidence-based practice. Nurse Educ 2005;30(3):127–32.
19. Academic ED SBIRT Research Collaborative. The impact of screening, brief intervention, and referral for treatment on emergency department patients' alcohol use. Ann Emerg Med 2007;50(6):699–710.
20. Desy PM, Perhats C. Alcohol screening, brief intervention, and referral in the emergency department: an implementation study. J Emerg Nurs 2008;34(1):11–9.
21. Beecroft PC, Dorey F, Wenten M. Turnover intention in new graduate nurses: a multivariate analysis. J Adv Nurs 2008;62(1):41–52.
22. Erenstein CF, McCaffrey BC. How healthcare work environments influence nurse retention. Holist Nurs Pract 2007;21(6):303–7.

A Collaborative Approach to Building the Capacity for Research and Evidence-Based Practice in Community Hospitals

Barbara B. Brewer, PhD, RN, MALS, MBA[a],*,
Melanie A. Brewer, DNSc, RN, FNP-BC[b], Alyce A. Schultz, RN, PhD, FAAN[c]

KEYWORDS
- Evidence-based practice • Models • Staff nurses

The use of best evidence to support nursing practice and the generation of new knowledge to use in practice are the hallmarks of excellence across the nation and the globe. Studies, however, continue to find that nurses at the bedside are limited in the resources and knowledge necessary to change the traditional nursing culture to one in which the use of evidence is incorporated into daily care.[1]

In the hectic world of today's nurse, the time needed to explore clinical and administrative questions systematically often is usurped by the ever-increasing demands of patient care and the work environment. In an effort to implement short-term solutions, quick fixes are put into practice as nurses focus on the "domain of action," continuing with traditional and multiple patterns of practice or, alternately, using a single article or hearsay to change practice, rather than focusing on the "domain of enduring change" by creating changes in attitudes and beliefs (eg, learning skills necessary to make organizational changes).[2] Creating and sustaining a learning environment in which point-of-care providers have the resources and knowledge necessary to improve patient outcomes through the use of best evidence focuses on the domain of enduring

[a] John C. Lincoln North Mountain Hospital, 250 E. Dunlap Avenue, Phoenix, AZ 85020, USA
[b] Nursing Research, Scottsdale Healthcare, 9003 E. Shea Boulevard, Scottsdale, AZ 85260, USA
[c] EBP Concepts, Alyce A. Schultz & Associates, LLC, 5747 W. Drake Court, Chandler, AZ 85226, USA
* Corresponding author.
E-mail address: barbara.brewer@jcl.com (B.B. Brewer).

Nurs Clin N Am 44 (2009) 11–25
doi:10.1016/j.cnur.2008.10.003
0029-6465/08/$ – see front matter © 2009 Elsevier Inc. All rights reserved.

change. Building the capacity and skills for evidence-based practice (EBP) at the point of care provides a long-term solution to changing patterns of thinking and promotes evidence-based care.

In its first 12 years of existence, a unique program designed to build the research capacity of point-of-care providers resulted in 16 publications co-authored by staff nurses, more than 40 posters, and 50 paper and symposium presentations at local, regional, national, and international conferences by staff nurses, recognition by nine professional nursing societies, including the Innovation in Clinical Excellence award from Sigma Theta Tau International and *Nursing Spectrum*, and three internal and four external grants.[3] The Clinical Scholarship resource paper first published by Sigma Theta Tau International in 1999 provided the overarching principles for the development of the Clinical Scholar Model (CSM) (**Fig. 1**).[4]

DEVELOPMENT OF THE CLINICAL SCHOLAR MODEL

The role of a clinically focused nurse researcher is to mentor nurses in the conduct and use of research and other forms of evidence. Since its inception in 1993, the clinical nursing research program at Maine Medical Center, a tertiary care hospital with more than 600 beds in northern New England, has promoted the professional growth of curious and creative direct-care nurses through education and mentorship by the nurse researcher on the conduct of research and the use of evidence in practice. Clinical nurses who already were asking clinical questions and wanting to change the way they currently were practicing were the first participants; they were eager to learn how to critique the research literature and integrate their findings to improve patient care. The practice of research utilization evolved to incorporating all forms of evidence when determining changes in nursing practice. The definition of EBP, adapted from the work of Stetler,[5] as used in the program, was

> the interdisciplinary approach to health care practice that bases decisions and practice strategies on the best available evidence including research findings, quality improvement data, clinical expertise, and patient values; considering feasibility, risk or harm, and costs.

External evidence is provided by empiric studies. Internal evidence may be data from quality improvement projects, program evaluations, satisfaction surveys, risk management, and other sources. These data are integrated and synthesized through the lens of clinical experts and are applied based on patient and family values and preferences. In nursing, implementing and sustaining EBP usually requires an organizational change and always requires the support and flexibility of management.

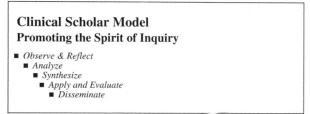

Fig. 1. The Clinical Scholar Model. (*Data from* STTI Resource Paper, 1999; and *Courtesy of* Alyce A. Schultz, RN, PhD, FAAN, Chandler, AZ.)

The CSM is an inductive model for mentoring point-of-care providers in the conduct of research and the implementation of evidence, diffusing EBP into the culture, and creating an organizational change in the work environment. The clinical questions are conceived by nurses at the bedside; using their questions as the context, the nurses are taught to find, critique, synthesize, and implement the evidence into their practice. The CSM facilitates responsibility and accountability for all nurses to base their care on evidence. It is decentralized, is predicated on "building a community of EBP mentors at the bedside," and fully supports the notion that for research to be translated into practice effectively, it must be read, understood, and valued by the direct-care provider.

Clinical scholarship promotes changing one's way of thinking from a task orientation to one of inquiry, reflection, and critical thinking.[4] Clinical scholarship does not mean that nurses must always be conducting research and publishing their findings, but it does mean that nurses must always be questioning their practice. Accordingly, clinical proficiency is not the same as clinical scholarship: performing a task consistently based on a written procedure does not make it scholarly unless the nurse questions whether the procedure needs to be performed in the first place.[4] Clinical scholars are innovators, the "out-of-the-box" thinkers who are always questioning their practice and who use their knowledge and the research to provide, teach, and manage patient care, based on knowledge rather than the rules. They seek information from multiple sources, continuously look for new sources of knowledge, and reflect on this information in planning the most effective care. They never stop asking "why?" They recognize that although their years of experience provide expertise in their area, there always is new information on the horizon, and that new information must be synthesized with the traditional ways of performing care.

Clinical scholarship requires strong skills in observation, analysis of varying forms of data, synthesis of the data/findings from all sources of evidence, application and evaluation of the synthesized results in practice, and dissemination of the information and sharing it with others so that the efforts are not duplicated needlessly in similar practice arenas. Each of these areas of the CSM was used to develop and refine the Clinical Scholar Program.

THE CLINICAL SCHOLAR PROGRAM

The Clinical Scholar Program is based on the CSM. The program is a series of six or seven workshops designed to build the capacity of nurses and other point-of-care providers in conducting research and in using research and other forms of evidence in practice.

Observation and Reflection

By using observation and reflection in their daily work, point-of-care providers can recognize patient responses to treatment and the cues that suggest that current practice is not effective. By cultivating these observational skills, Clinical scholars move beyond just observation to asking the important clinical questions. Other prompts that might generate researchable clinical questions include changes in quality outcome or risk management data, scorecard reports, knowledge shared by a new staff member, new knowledge learned at a conference, family concerns about a particular patient's response to a nursing or interdisciplinary intervention, or new regulatory requirements for reducing nurse-sensitive patient outcomes. Ultimately, the question is written in the population of interest/intervention of interest/comparative intervention/outcome (PICO) format. The scholar then completes a library search for articles addressing the intervention/innovation, outcomes, or both.

Analysis and Critique

The scholars learn to critique the various types of research designs, including qualitative studies, quantitative studies, and meta-analyses. The important components of a study are put into an evaluation table, including, if appropriate, the statistical outcomes that relate to the intervention or outcome of interest. It is important to be able to differentiate quickly between published articles that are and are not research. The purpose of this learning is to prepare the scholars to synthesize all the evidence later and determine its strength to support practice changes. These workshops include methods of searching for and evaluating published guidelines and systematic reviews. The scholars also begin the process of identifying sources of internal data for baseline data collection and ultimately for monitoring continuous improvement of outcomes.

Synthesis of the Evidence

Synthesis of the internal and external evidence is critical in determining whether the evidence is strong enough to change practice without increasing risk or harm to the patients, to improve outcomes without significantly increasing the costs of care, and to determine the feasibility of implementation in the practice setting. The strength of the evidence is determined through amalgamation of the study designs, the statistical and clinical relevance of the findings, the quality of study methods, and the consistency of the results across studies. The findings are put in synthesis tables that clearly show the reliability of study outcomes based on similar interventions. Multiple synthesis tables may be required to answer a single clinical question, depending on how interventions have been applied and outcomes have been defined.

Application and Evaluation

The synthesized results are used to develop or change a clinical guideline, policy, procedure, or pathway. Throughout the process, attention is paid to team development, team membership, and consideration of challenges that may inhibit implementation of the new ideas. In this phase of the CSM, a pilot implementation plan is developed that addresses the need to educate nonmembers of the project or study team, to plan for systematic data collection, and to assure fidelity of the intervention. Outcome data form the basis for adopting the new practice throughout a facility or system, for discarding the new practice, or for adapting and re-evaluating the practice further before adoption.

Dissemination

A research study or an evidence-based practice change is not complete until the results have been disseminated to a professional audience, either through presentation, publication, or both. The last workshop addresses writing an abstract for poster or podium presentation, followed by a day of presentations to the administrators and other point-of-care providers in the facility. The projects and studies are presented at their point of progress.

THE FIRST CLINICAL SCHOLAR PROGRAM

The first Clinical Scholar Program was conducted in at Maine Medical Center by a cadre of 10 staff nurse and clinical nurse specialist innovators who had worked with the model explicitly and implicitly for almost a decade. Fifty nurses started the six-part series, and 45 nurses (90%) completed the program. Fourteen clinically focused projects were developed. Of these 14 projects, 10 were completed, and eight have been presented at local, regional, national, and international conferences. One nurse was recognized for her study by the American Nephrology Nurses Association in 2005. All the original Clinical Scholar facilitators have completed a master's degree or currently are enrolled in a graduate program.

Collaboration, Cooperation, and Accomplishments

The Clinical Scholar Program is the format for EBP and research fellowships in multiple settings. The successes and challenges in a community hospital and a freestanding pediatric hospital are described here.

Building Evidence-Based Practice Capacity in a Community Hospital

John C. Lincoln North Mountain Hospital (JCLNMH) is a 266-bed community hospital with a Level I trauma center. It was the first hospital in Phoenix, AZ to receive Magnet designation. The hospital is part of a health network containing two hospitals, physician practices, and a longstanding mission to the community, demonstrated through multiple social and health services incorporated in the Desert Mission, which is the social service division of the network.

Nursing leadership began building its capacity for EBP as part of its Magnet journey. Evidence was incorporated into policies, procedures, and protocols, but many still contained textbook references and manufacturer guidelines as their only sources of evidence. Additionally, there were minimal levels of nursing research and quality Improvement activities. Many nurses were long tenured in the organization and had received their nursing education more than a decade earlier. As a result, there was confusion regarding the components of EBP and minimal, if any, experience using computer-based databases for locating relevant literature.

Leadership recognized that transforming the organizational culture to embrace evidence as a way of informing daily patient care would require further knowledge and skill development in the nursing staff, accessibility to evidence resources at the point of care, and the commitment of financial resources in the form of dedicated time for study and project work. Furthermore, leadership recognized the need to accelerate the pace for transformation to build a cadre of nurses who could help to promote and implement research and EBP.

Recognition of the need to accelerate the pace of transformation was not enough to change practice. Moving forward was limited by the educational level of the nursing staff, which primarily was at the associate degree level. Only 30% of direct-care nurses were prepared at the baccalaureate level. Many of the nurses had been educated before the advent of computer-based databases. As a result, nurses had limited skills in searching, critiquing, and synthesizing literature. Few of the nursing staff were prepared at the master's level, so it was not possible to mentor less-skilled staff by drawing on internal expertise. The staff members who held master's degrees held managerial and educational positions.

Creative partnerships

Building capacity for EBP in bedside nurses requires individual skill development as well as leadership and an organizational culture that promotes and supports its use.[6] Melnyk[7] suggests that once excitement about learning and applying new skills related to EBP wanes, the presence of mentors may support sustainability of EBP within an organization. Nursing leadership at JCLNMH was committed to improving nursing staff skills in EBP. Building skills and providing staff support fell within the responsibilities of the director of professional practice, who was a doctorally prepared nurse researcher. The director, newly hired in mid-2005, was accountable for nursing research, EBP, and oversight of the Magnet program. She had the skills to find and evaluate evidence for practice and was comfortable providing content to staff nurses. She felt a sense of urgency to accelerate the transformation of the culture from tradition based to evidence based. As a result, she thought it prudent to find a model that could be used to define the curriculum and reduce the time needed for content development. The JCLNMH was fortunate to be located near a university with faculty who were internationally known for their expertise in EBP; therefore she investigated options for adjunct faculty opportunities while learning more about potential resources and support from the university.

Faculty at Arizona State University had developed two EBP models, Advancing Research and Clinical Practice through Close Collaboration (ARCC) and the CSM, both of which are built on mentors who facilitate the diffusion of EBP through an organization. A major difference between the two models is that Melnyk and Fineout-Overholt's ARCC model uses advanced-practice nurses as mentors, whereas Schultz' Clinical Scholar Model uses bedside nursing staff as mentors.[8] The CSM was better suited to the limited number of advanced-practice nurses within the JCLNMH.

About this time, an opportunity arose that facilitated the development of a creative partnership between the hospital and the university. The university recently had developed an EBP post-master's certificate program. One of the courses in the program was an online course in outcomes management, which was an area of expertise of the hospital's nurse researcher. A partnership was formed through which the hospital's nurse researcher taught the outcomes course for the university, and in exchange the university provided a series of workshops taught by a faculty member. The partnership was of benefit to both parties: the hospital enjoyed the university faculty's expertise, and the university enjoyed the expertise of the hospital's nurse researcher, without exchanging money. The nurse researcher invited the developer of the CSM to present information about projects completed by bedside nurses. Nurses who attended the presentation were excited. Many had questions, began thinking of ideas they could investigate, and wanted more information. Most of the individuals who composed the first cohort of scholars attended this session.

Developing content and setting expectations

Once the partnership had been established, the content, dates, and times for the workshops were developed jointly. Most of the workshops were based on the CSM, but content regarding change theory was added. Change theory was incorporated to provide tools nurses could use to introduce practice changes and obtain support for the practice changes from other staff. As noted earlier, these practice changes require organizational changes that many staff nurses never have orchestrated.

Once the dates and content for workshops had been determined, expectations for clinical scholars and nursing leadership were established. An EBP fellowship was established by the nurse researcher, who acted as the mentor for all fellows. In collaboration with members of the Clinical Research Committee, an application for the fellowship was developed that asked about the applicant's education level, exposure to EBP projects, and ideas for potential projects. Selection criteria for the fellowship also were discussed with members of the committee. Two selection criteria were recommended: all applicants must be in good disciplinary standing and must hold a minimum of a bachelor's degree. The goal was to begin with a cohort of 10 to 15 fellows.

Nurses interested in applying for the fellowship were given a list of the expectations they would be required to meet if selected. All fellows were expected to attend all workshops, to complete a project, and to submit an abstract to a conference. Nursing leadership had agreed to give each fellow 12 hours of paid release time during the pay period of the workshop. Fellows could use the time to attend the workshop and complete individual or group work on their projects. To date two cohorts of fellows have completed the Clinical Scholar series of workshops. The following sections summarize the experience for each cohort.

The first cohort

Information about the fellowship was shared with clinical directors, members of shared leadership, charge nurses, and through fliers distributed to all nursing units. Twenty-three staff nurses, clinical educators, and clinical directors completed applications. Ten of the applicants had earned a bachelor's or master's degree in nursing science, three held bachelor's degrees in areas other than nursing, one held a non-nursing master of science degree, and five held an associate degree in nursing. Four of the applicants who held an associate's degree were pursuing a bachelor's degree in nursing. Rather than turn away applicants who were excited about the possibility of developing new skills in EBP, all were accepted into the fellowship. Of the 23 accepted, 21 began the fellowship. Two nurses dropped out before the first session because they could not commit to attending all workshops. Nineteen nurses completed the series.

The fellows were from four hospital units: two critical care units, a medical unit, and a medical-surgical unit. Although unplanned, the limited number of units resulted in common project interests among the fellows, greater accessibility to discuss progress and ideas among themselves between workshops, and increased visibility on their units of the fellows'excitement in gaining new skills in clinical inquiry.

From the start, the fellows were full of enthusiasm for the new skills they were gaining. The energy levels during the workshops were palpable. With each workshop, the level of dialogue increased. Scholars discussed such things as the literature they were or were not finding, changes being made to their questions as they delved more deeply into the literature, their surprise regarding the limited availability of research for many of their topics, and the positive responses they were experiencing on their units as they shared what they were learning with the other staff. **Table 1** contains project information for the two cohorts that have completed Clinical Scholar workshops. Projects generally focused on improving care for patient populations admitted to the units represented by the fellows.

The second cohort

During the fall of 2007, fellowships began for the second cohort of scholars. Applications were distributed using the same process as with the first cohort. Interest continued to be high and resulted in 22 applications from staff nurses, clinical educators, and clinical directors. All applicants began the workshops; 18 completed the series. Fellows in the second cohort were from obstetrics, medical, medical-surgical, surgical, perioperative services, and critical care units. Unlike the first cohort, half of whom were critical care nurses, the second cohort contained only one critical care nurse. Educational levels were mixed; as happened in the first group, those who had had previous exposure to research courses or literature searches helped those who were less

Table 1
Summary of John C. Lincoln North Mountain Hospital clinical scholar program projects

Cohort	Specialty	Project
1	Critical care	Effect of ambient music versus headphones on stress in patients after coronary artery bypass graft
1	Critical care	Effect of chlorhexidine oral care on reducing ventilator associated pneumonia
1	Critical care	Use of an EBP protocol to standardize care and reduce pulmonary complications in patients after coronary artery bypass graft
1	Critical care	Understanding nurse barriers to using EBP protocols to reduce the prevalence of pressure ulcers in critical care patients
1	Medicine/surgery	Reducing falls in hospitalized patients
1	Medicine/surgery	Using Caring Theory to improve work environment for nurses
2	Medicine/surgery	Methods of cross-contamination of *Clostridium difficile* in hospitals
2	Medicine/surgery	Evidence-based smoking cessation intervention for nurses
2	Obstetrics	Using chart audits to change practice in nursing staff
2	Medicine/surgery	Reducing musculoskeletal injuries in nursing staff
2	Medicine/surgery	Effect of a centralized orientation unit on sense of belonging and satisfaction of new graduate nurses
2	Medicine/surgery	Predictors of readmission within 30 days of patients who have community-acquired pneumonia

experienced. To a person, regardless of educational level and prior experience, fellows reported that they learned new information from the workshops and felt much more confident about their skills.

Based on feedback received from the first cohort, changes were made in the spacing between workshops and the emphasis placed on some topics. Workshops for the first cohort were not spaced apart evenly but were spaced to allow more time for evaluating and synthesizing evidence. Two months were planned to provide balance with reading articles, work, and school schedules for many fellows. Participants recommended allowing less time in the future because they felt they lost momentum during the long interval between sessions. They also reported that they tended to leave homework until close to the next session, so having more time between sessions was not helpful. As with the first series, most of the workshops were taught by the faculty member, searching was taught by the hospital librarian, and change theory was taught by the hospital's nurse researcher, who served as the mentor for all projects.

Scholars from the first cohort served as support for the second group. They reported their experiences and the progress they were making on their projects. When the second cohort began meeting, projects from the first group were at different stages of maturity. In fact, projects ranged from being ready for institutional review board approval to a change in topic requiring beginning a new search for literature.

Challenges and solutions
One of the challenges faced with both cohorts was maintaining momentum between workshops. As stated earlier, some slowing of momentum was related to the length of the interval between workshops. Some was related to the inability of group members to schedule time to work together and the inherent frustration caused by scheduling

difficulties. As with any group, different members had different levels of energy for the project work and different levels of commitment involving other aspects in their lives, such as family or school assignments. Some groups were better able than others to find ways to work together productively.

Another challenge involved providing support for those who had steeper learning curves. Despite frequent offers by the nurse researcher to provide help to those who were having difficulty with searching, evaluating, or synthesizing literature, few individuals in the first cohort asked for help. As a result, time was not always used efficiently when groups did meet, and progress on projects slowed. In an attempt to avoid this situation with the second cohort, more structure was added to the fellowship. Project groups were asked to meet with the nurse researcher between workshops covering evaluation and synthesis of the literature and to review their evaluation and synthesis tables with the nurse researcher so problems could be identified and resolved in a more timely way.

The development of synthesis tables was difficult to master and problematic for all individuals in both cohorts. Fellows tended to summarize their evaluation tables rather than integrate them into a synthesis of all evidence. A technique that helped the second cohort clarify where there was misunderstanding was the use of workshop time to review preselected articles together. Attendees were asked to work within their groups to develop a synthesis table for each outcome addressed in the articles. They were asked to specify how each outcome was measured and to evaluate whether measurement was consistent across studies. They then were asked to synthesize the evidence for each outcome. Tables were reviewed as a group so everyone could see how to synthesize correctly the evidence provided in the articles. The exercise worked so well that the first cohort was scheduled for a "booster" workshop in which they repeated this process. Again, attendees found the exercise very useful in identifying where they did not understand how to distill information from multiple studies into a cogent recommendation for practice change based on the strength and quality of the evidence.

Group process issues plagued project teams in both cohorts. This program may have been the first time that some nurses had worked in this type of group situation. Some nurses were better than others in dealing with group conflicts and resolving issues among group members. Some groups were able to divide the work by assigning pieces to each group member; others believed each member should do each part. Based on the experiences of the first two cohorts, a workshop taught by experts in organizational development and containing content on group process, managing group conflict, assigning workload, and similar issues will be added to the next series of workshops.

Personal and organizational outcomes

Nurses who completed the series of workshops gained confidence in asking relevant clinical questions, searching literature for best evidence, critiquing research articles, critiquing systematic reviews and published guidelines, and synthesizing multiple sources of evidence on a topic. Many have stated that what they have learned has made them feel more empowered in their own practice and more confident of their ability to find answers to their questions. Some have incorporated information from internal evidence into the way they personally manage patients.[9]

As noted earlier, many of the participants were in school during the time they attended the Clinical Scholar workshops. One participant, who also was a member of the clinical research committee, decided to return to school to obtain her bachelor's degree because she was concerned that she would not be accepted to participate in the fellowship unless she did. She had ignored the recommendation of her nurse manager on multiple previous occasions but changed her mind once she feared she would miss the opportunity to be part of the fellowship.[10] Three members of the first cohort decided to return to school for master's degrees as a result of their participation in the fellowship. Several members of both cohorts currently are in school pursuing master's degrees.

As a condition of participation, fellows agreed to prepare and submit abstracts to conferences. To date, five abstracts have been submitted by fellows. Two were accepted for podium presentations at national conferences,[9,11] and three have been submitted for consideration for an upcoming conference. It was the first time any of the staff nurses had presented at a conference. Each year the hospital presents a series of exemplar awards to nurses during Nurses' Week. In 2007, one of the nurses selected for a podium presentation was recognized with the Student of the Year exemplar; in 2008, a different nurse presenter was recognized with the EBP and Research exemplar.

Organizational outcomes include multiple research and EBP projects that will improve patient outcomes and the work environment for nurses. A second outcome has been recognition of the investment the organization has made in its nursing staff. Information about the program and the experience of participants has been reported in *NurseWeek*, *American Nurse*, and at a national Magnet conference. Nursing leadership is proud of the accomplishments and will continue to invest in the program.

The Clinical Scholar Program in a Children's Hospital

In an effort to build capacity to deliver safe, high-quality health care to acutely ill infants and children, nursing leadership at Phoenix Children's Hospital, a 300-bed pediatric hospital, determined that a practical approach was needed to create an environment of evidence-based care (EBC). Executive leadership fully supported advancing evidence-based decision making in clinical practice across disciplines. The need to improve outcomes for patients and families was well recognized among bedside care providers, and several were eager to discover new strategies to improve care. Most bedside clinicians rarely accessed the available online library resources or contacted the medical librarian, however, and many were unaware of the existence of the medical library. The first step toward improving outcomes required educating bedside clinicians in finding and using the best available clinical and scientific evidence for practice.

Phoenix Children's Hospital recently had expanded from "a hospital within a hospital" to a freestanding 300-bed facility. Establishment of the nursing leadership team and of policies and guidelines for practice and the development of a complete staff for each unit were well underway. Approximately 23% of the nurses in the institution held a bachelor's degree or higher. These factors supported the need for EBC and also created challenges for implementation in a new facility.

During her faculty interview at a local university, an internationally recognized expert in EBP and the developer of the CSM presented "Creating the Spirit of Inquiry Using the Clinical Scholar Model." Her presentation and the discussion that followed resonated with bedside nurses and with the nursing leadership team. The CSM provided a framework for (1) educating nurses and other care providers to find, critically appraise, synthesize, implement, and evaluate the best evidence for practice, (2) conducting research when no evidence was available, which often is the case in pediatric and neonatal care, (3) disseminating findings, and (4) creating a cadre of mentors to encourage the spread of evidence-based skills and knowledge to improve outcomes.[3] Nursing leadership and bedside nurses chose the CSM as a roadmap to excellence for the care of children and their families.

Collaboration with university faculty

A collaborative partnership was established with a college of nursing at a local university to support implementation of the CSM. The partnership involved a joint appointment for three individuals (two nursing faculty from the university, each with 25% appointment at the hospital, and a faculty appointment for the hospital's nurse researcher at 50% time) to complete the one full-time nursing research position supported by the hospital. The faculty included the developer of the CSM and an expert in neonatal clinical care and research. In year two of the partnership, the neonatal faculty member accepted a faculty position out of state, and subsequently the partnership included one faculty member and the nurse researcher. The neonatal faculty member has continued to support projects at the hospital with neonatal nurses.

The joint appointment model was chosen to implement the CSM in this clinical environment for several reasons. Leadership at Phoenix Children's Hospital and at Arizona State University had begun to develop collaborative partnerships for advancing pediatric nursing education and for research. The Chief Nurse Executive for the hospital was enthusiastic about the opportunity to have an EBP expert as part of the nursing research team, and, with the Dean of the College of Nursing, established an agreement to exchange faculty time for teaching and mentored research opportunities for the nurse researcher, which would enhance further opportunities for bedside clinicians to participate in relevant clinical nursing research. Funding for one full-time equivalent position was paid to the university in exchange for the faculty collaboration.

Program implementation

The Clinical Scholars Program, based on the CSM, was initiated at the hospital in 2005. Information on the program was presented to all bedside clinicians (nurses, respiratory therapists, pharmacists, and other allied health providers) who held bachelor's or master's degrees. This decision was based on the assumption that persons with a bachelor's degree would have taken a research course and basic statistics. The EBP faculty member led the Clinical Scholars Program workshops at the hospital. All three program faculty met with new clinical scholars as they developed and implemented projects. The diverse backgrounds of the faculty supported the scholars in a variety of interest areas.

Scholar selection process

Initially, the selection of the scholars occurred through individual expression of interest via an e-mail to the nurse researcher with a signed statement of support from their unit manager. Participants were selected if they committed to attend each of the six workshops in addition to the time required to complete assignments following the workshop (eg, reading the articles, searching for evidence, conducting evidence appraisal and synthesis, participating in group discussion, and project development). The responsibility for requesting time away from clinical care to participate in each workshop and to complete assignments belonged to the individual scholar. Unfortunately, several participants missed workshops because of scheduling conflicts and lack of staff to cover bedside patient care needs. Additional time for team meetings and project development outside of the workshops was rarely possible.

The selection process has evolved with each successive workshop series to the current formal application process. The application, adapted from JCLNMH, includes (1) a description of the potential scholar's interest in and expected outcomes for participation in the program; (2) area of interest for an EBP project with inclusion of a PICO question; (3) a letter of support from the unit manager including confirmation of release time for workshop attendance and time required to work on the proposed project (8 hours of workshop participation and 4 hours of reading/review time); and (4) a statement signed by the participant confirming agreement to prepare for and attend all workshops. Potential scholars complete and submit the application packet for review by the faculty approximately 1 month before the beginning of the program. Selection is based on successful completion of the packet. Preference is given to applicants who have completed a bachelor's degree, but no applicant has been denied entry to the program because of educational level. The number of scholars in any workshop series is limited to 20.

Program mentors
Initially, five master's and one doctorally prepared nurse met with program faculty to discuss their role as mentors for the scholars. Each expressed interest in and commitment to helping facilitate the program and mentor bedside clinicians in the processes of EBP and research. Unfortunately, most were unable to participate in the program because of lack of available time away from their clinical roles. One neonatal nurse practitioner attended four of the workshops and, together with the other faculty, supported the development of a research study in the neonatal ICU (NICU).

The first workshop series
Scholars participating in the first series of workshops were from various disciplines and educational backgrounds, including associate's degree, bachelor's and master's prepared nurses, bachelor's prepared dieticians, associate's degree and master's prepared respiratory therapists, and a pharmacy intern. The clinical scholars worked in teams with shared interest areas whenever possible. The topic and PICO question chosen were negotiated among the group members. Of the initial 22 participants, 10 completed the program, including one dietician and nine nurses. Various reasons were given for lack of participation, but most were related to the requirements of their clinical roles. Specifically, the need to work overtime in the winter months, lack of staff coverage to enable participants to take the time away from the care unit, and last-minute schedule changes caused by colleagues' illness contributed to absenteeism.

The first series of seven all-day workshops were held semi-monthly. This format was based on previous experience with implementation of the Clinical Scholar Program at another hospital. The timeframe between workshops may have been too long to support momentum and interest, because most participants did not complete reading assignments or work together in their groups between sessions. Additionally, management support seemed to decrease between workshops. Communication with the scholars was challenging, because e-mail was not consistently available to all employees during this time.

Despite the challenges, the first series of workshops led to further discussion and awareness of the need for evidence to guide practice. Three scholars who completed the program presented posters or podium presentations at national symposia, and one presented at an international conference the next year. A randomized, controlled trial implemented by NICU staff and including the initial team of nurses, dieticians, and the neonatal faculty member, is still in progress. Other successes include the testimonials of the clinical scholars about their experiences in the program as they encouraged other staff to participate. Nursing leadership and management also noted motivation and additional interest among staff in asking clinical questions about their practice.

The second workshop series
The second workshop series differed from the first in several respects. Selection occurred through an application process, as described previously. Scholars in the

second series were attending either a Registered Nurse-Bachelor of Science in Nursing program or a master's program with pediatric or neonatal nurse practitioner coursework. The timeframe between workshops was shortened to 6 weeks, and an additional workshop was held at the end of the series to assist scholars with abstract writing. Of the 18 scholars who began the program, 16 completed it. Although attendance during the second series was significantly better than in the first series, obtaining release time to complete reading assignments and work on projects with team members was still a challenge. Manager support for workshop participation and project development increased in most clinical areas but continued to lag in others.

After program completion, the clinical scholars continued to work on their projects. Two groups have initiated research studies, and three evidence-based projects have been initiated. Interest in conducting EBC has continued to escalate among scholars who have completed the program in terms of discussions with peers, in encouraging others to participate in the Clinical Scholars Program, and in searching for and using evidence to guide practice.

The third workshop series

The format of the third workshop series was seven 8-hour workshops held monthly with additional time for discussion of project development so that the scholars might share ideas and learn from the work of their colleagues. Most of the workshop content was didactic presentation and discussion regarding the principles and practice of finding, appraising, synthesizing, applying, and measuring the best available internal and external evidence. Preparation for project implementation, including presentation to the institutional review board by the scholars, was a key component. Of the 10 bedside nurses and nurse educators who began the program, 9 nurses recently completed it. The clinical scholars had baccalaureate degrees or currently were enrolled in a Registered Nurse-Bachelor of Science in Nursing program. **Table 2** summarizes examples of the projects initiated or completed by the clinical scholars for each series of workshops.

Program outcomes and conclusions

Through collaboration with Arizona State University and EBP experts, the Clinical Scholars Program has been successful in enhancing the use of evidence to guide practice at Phoenix Children's Hospital. In addition to improving outcomes for patients and families through the use of evidence in practice, those who have completed the program have begun to mentor others in beginning to question their current practice. The nurses and dietician who completed the program have graduated from bachelor's and master's programs, and two have been accepted in doctoral programs.

The clinical scholars have participated in events at the hospital to highlight program outcomes, including Nursing Grand Rounds and podium and poster presentations during Nurses' Week. In addition, scholars have submitted proposals and made presentations to the hospital institutional review board. One scholar now is participating in a national collaborative to study best practices related to risk assessment and prevention of falling. Scholars who have completed the program have initiated journal clubs (oncology and NICU), and nine have submitted or presented their work at regional, national, and international conferences. These presentations illustrate how bedside clinicians can use evidence and develop different ways of thinking and questioning clinical practice. The Clinical Scholars Program has been successful in leading the effort to change the delivery of clinical practice to enhance both the quality and safety of health care for children in the Southwest.

Table 2
Summary of Phoenix Children's Hospital clinical scholar program projects

Series	Specialty	Project
1	Neonatal	Effects of holding infants during gavage feeding
1	Medicine/surgery	Development of an evidence-based pediatric guideline for assessing risk and preventing falls
2	Airway	Evaluation of an evidence-based car seat challenge test for children on ventilators
2	Pediatric ICU	Evaluation of an evidence-based sedation protocol for critically ill children
2	Neonatal ICU	Evaluation of an evidence-based ventilator-associated pneumonia protocol
2	Emergency	Descriptive study of Zofran and oral fluid therapy for children who have acute gastroenteritis
2	Oncology	Implementation of a symptom management checklist for children with cancer
3	Oncology	Phenomenologic study of the educational experience of parents of children who have acute lymphocytic leukemia
3	Neonatal ICU	Evidence-based protocol for administering low dose medications in low birth weight infants
3	Oncology	Discussion of fertility options by oncology providers
3	Pulmonary	Outcomes of patient education
3	Emergency	Personal protective equipment compliance in the emergency department

CONCLUSIONS AND IMPLICATIONS FOR PRACTICE AND RESEARCH

Practicing as a clinical scholar distinguishes a job from a career in nursing. To sustain excellence, clinicians must be involved actively in the selection and collection of quality improvement data and the critique and synthesis of evidence. Collaboration among multiple disciplines is paramount for the decision making necessary for clinical research and EBP. Involvement in the Clinical Scholar Program has renewed the spirit of nursing. A translational research study is planned to evaluate the outcomes of the CSM as compared with the usual methods for promoting the spirit of inquiry.

ACKNOWLEDGMENT

The authors acknowledge the support of the Department of Nursing at Maine Medical Center, Portland, ME during the development and early implementation of the Clinical Scholar Model. The collaborative efforts in the community hospitals would not have been possible without the vision of the Dean at Arizona State University, College of Nursing and Healthcare Innovation, and the chief nurse executives, nursing managers, and nursing colleagues within the direct-care settings.

REFERENCES

1. Pravikoff DS, Tanner AB, Pierce ST. Readiness of U.S. nurses for evidence-based practice: many don't understand or value research and have had little or no training to help them find evidence on which to base their practice. Am J Nurs 2005; 105(9):40–52.

2. Senge PM. The fifth discipline: the art and practice of the learning organization. 1st edition. New York: Doubleday/Currency; 1990.
3. Schultz AA. Clinical scholars at the bedside: an EBP mentorship model for today. Excellence in Nursing Knowledge; 2005. p. 4–11.
4. Clinical scholarship task force: clinical scholarship resource paper. Available at: http://www.nursingsociety.org/aboutus/Documents/clinical_scholarship_paper.pdf. Accessed June 3, 2008.
5. Stetler CB. Updating the stetler model of research utilization to facilitate evidence-based practice. Nurs Outlook 2001;49(6):272–9.
6. Rycroft-Malone JO. Evidence-informed practice: from individual to context. J Nurs Manag 2008;16:404–8.
7. Melnyk BM. The evidence-based practice mentor: a promising strategy for implementing and sustaining EBP in healthcare systems. Worldviews of Evidence Based Nursing 2007;4:123–5.
8. Fineout-Overholt E, Melnyk BM, Schultz A. Transforming health care from the inside out: advancing evidence-based practice in the 21st century. J Prof Nurs 2005;21(6):335–44.
9. Alber D, Brewer BB, Berkley C, et al. 2008. Collection and analysis of fall risk characteristics in hospitalized adults. Presented at the Ninth Annual EBP Conference. Glendale (AZ), February 14, 2008.
10. Ratner T. Evidence-based practice 101. Available at: http://include.nurse.com/apps/pbcs.dll/article?AID=/20080114/SW02/80111033. Accessed May 30, 2008.
11. Brewer BB, Schultz AA, George N, et al. 2007. A community hospital's path to bedside nurse competence in EBP. Presented at the Eleventh National Magnet Conference. Atlanta (GA), October 5, 2007.

Development of an Evidence-Based Practice and Research Collaborative Among Urban Hospitals

Susan Mace Weeks, MS, RN, CNS-P/MH, LMFT, LCDC[a],*,
June Marshall, RN, MS, NEA-BC[b], Paulette Burns, PhD, RN[c]

KEYWORDS

- Evidence-based practice • Research • Collaboration
- Nursing research • Community partnerships

The Texas Christian University (TCU) Center for Evidence-Based Practice and Research (CEBPR) was established in the Harris College of Nursing and Health Sciences in June, 2006. Originally funded by an internal TCU grant, the CEBPR was developed as a point of connection between nursing faculty members and the clinical agencies where student practicum experiences occur. There was a growing focus on evidence-based practice and research occurring among the area hospitals, motivated largely by the hospitals' pursuit of the American Nurses Credentialing Center's Magnet designation. It was recognized that nursing faculty members had expertise in the areas of evidence-based practice and research that would be useful to hospitals focusing efforts in these realms.

One activity that occurred during the first year of the TCU CEBPR's existence was the sponsorship of an internationally recognized expert who has gained acclaim for her ability to engage direct-care nurses in both evidence-based practice and research. Dr. Alyce Schultz is known for her ability to create enthusiasm and commitment in the individuals to whom she speaks. She was invited to come to the TCU campus, and arrangements were made for her to present also at five area hospitals. Each hospital decided on the setting and the audience to whom she would speak and made arrangements to provide nursing continuing education credits. During a 3-day period, Dr. Schultz spoke to more than 500 nurses in the Dallas-Fort Worth area.

[a] Center for Evidence-Based Practice and Research, Texas Christian University, TCU Box 298620, Fort Worth, TX 76129, USA
[b] Center for Nurse Excellence, Medical City Hospital, 7777 Forest Lane, Dallas, TX 75230, USA
[c] Harris College of Nursing and Health Sciences, Texas Christian University, TCU Box 298625, Fort Worth, TX 76129, USA
* Corresponding author.
E-mail address: s.weeks@tcu.edu (S.M. Weeks).

Nurs Clin N Am 44 (2009) 27–31
doi:10.1016/j.cnur.2008.10.009
0029-6465/08/$ – see front matter © 2009 Elsevier Inc. All rights reserved.
nursing.theclinics.com

The director of the TCU CEBPR escorted Dr. Schultz to each of her speaking engagements. While traveling between two of the sites, they began to brainstorm ways to build on the enthusiasm that had developed during the presentations. One of the ideas that emerged from the discussion was the development of a collaborative of hospitals focused on evidence-based practice and research. From this idea, the TCU Evidence-Based Practice and Research (EBPR) Collaborative was born.

The initial goal of the TCU EBPR Collaborative was quite simple: to increase connections between area hospitals in an effort to increase evidence-based practice and research. One of the initial concerns was whether competing hospitals could collaborate effectively. Fortunately, that concern has not been a problem. The hospitals involved in the Collaborative have been very willing to share their successes and struggles. From the beginning, the Collaborative has been open to any individual or any agency wishing to participate. Announcements of meetings are distributed by e-mail, and recipients are encouraged to share the announcement with others. Within the first 6 months, nurses from 30 hospitals and three universities had become involved in the Collaborative.

ACTIVITIES

The first meeting of the TCU EBPR Collaborative was held in June, 2007. The hope was for an attendance of 10 to 15 individuals; in fact, more than 20 nurses attended. The first meeting was held on the TCU campus and was focused on sharing the idea of the Collaborative, sharing ideas of EBPR projects that seemed to be successful, and brainstorming future projects for the Collaborative.

The second meeting was held in August, 2007 at an area hospital that volunteered to host the meeting because of its central location between Dallas and Fort Worth. The attendance at this meeting increased to more than 40 individuals. During this meeting, each hospital was encouraged to describe a specific idea or project that had infused EBPR successfully in its practice setting. The projects described ranged from the situation, background, assessment, and request (SBAR) method of hand-off communication to a presentation titled "Pico de Practice" that focused on the population/intervention/comparison/outcome (PICO) method of formulating clinical questions. A highlight of the second meeting was a presentation by an intensive care staff nurse who shared how he had changed practice related to the use of oral-gastric tubes as a result of a clinical question he had investigated. Hearing the excitement of a staff nurse who had implemented an evidence-based practice change effectively was inspiring to the attendees.

At the end of the second meeting, a decision was made to form two taskforces from the Collaborative. One taskforce would focus on the development of a series of workshops and mentoring opportunities for direct-care nurses to increase their knowledge and skills related to evidence-based practice (referred to as an "EBP Fellowship"). The second taskforce would focus on joint research projects focusing broadly on "Research about Nurses." During October, 2007 both taskforces met on the TCU campus, and reports from these two meetings were given during the third meeting of the Collaborative, which occurred in November of 2007.

The third meeting also was held at a hospital centrally located between Dallas and Fort Worth. In addition to hearing from the two taskforces, additional sharing of EBPR projects and ideas occurred. The CEBPR director had conducted a brief survey among chief nursing officers (CNOs) of participating hospitals to assess their ability to provide salary and other financial support for an EBP Fellowship for direct-care nurses. The results of this survey were announced, and options based on the

CNOs' willingness to support the Fellowship were discussed. One specific idea that evolved from this meeting was the desire to host a CNO speaker from a Magnet-recognized hospital system. This CNO had made an earlier offer to the TCU Dean of Nursing and Health Sciences to speak at an area nursing event, and the Collaborative was excited to have this CNO share her thoughts about fostering and supporting evidence-based practice and research in a hospital setting. A decision was made to invite this CNO to speak at the next Collaborative meeting and to invite area CNOs to attend the meeting. The desired outcome was to learn from this Magnet CNO and to garner continued support among area CNOs for the activities of the TCU EBPR Collaborative.

In February 2008, Joyce Batcheller, CNO of the Seton Family of Hospitals in Austin, Texas, gave a presentation to the TCU EBPR Collaborative on the topic of "Resources to Support Evidence-Based Practice and Research in the Hospital Setting." More than 100 nurse leaders from hospitals in the Dallas-Fort Worth area attended the event. The event continued the excitement about promoting evidence-based practice and research in area hospitals and also helped the nurse leaders understand the human and financial resources needed to create a culture of evidence-based nursing practice.

CHALLENGES

The challenge initially thought most likely to be a problem for the TCU EBPR Collaborative, establishing cooperation among competitors, has not emerged as an issue of concern. Instead, each agency involved in the Collaborative has been willing to share ideas, support, and motivation with other Collaborative members. Perhaps the open, inclusive nature of the Collaborative has helped foster this spirit of sharing. Other challenges that have been faced are the distance between agencies and the ever-present challenge of communication. Both these challenges have been addressed by using electronic communication as the primary means of communication between meetings. An electronic distribution list is maintained by the TCU CEBPR, and notices are sent to Collaborative members through this electronic distribution list. TCU also has agreed to provide a Web-based portal that will allow members of the Collaborative to post and comment on shared documents and to post questions and ideas on a discussion board.

A potential challenge for the TCU EBPR Collaborative was addressed successfully through open communication. The area hospital trade organization (Dallas-Fort Worth Hospital Council, DFWHC) decided to form a group of nurse researchers focused on joint research a few months after the beginning of the TCU Collaborative. The announcement of the DFWHC nursing research group was sent to nurse researchers in area hospitals, many of whom already were involved in the TCU Collaborative. Several of the nurse researchers who received the DFWHC announcement expressed their desire to remain committed to the TCU Collaborative and focused on the projects currently being developed rather than participating in a separate initiative. As the organizer of the TCU Collaborative, the TCU CEBPR director was included on the replies that several of the nurse researchers sent to the DFWHC organizers and quickly reached out to the DFWHC organizers to invite their involvement in the TCU Collaborative. The DFWHC was supportive of the TCU Collaborative and, after an initial meeting to explore interest, decided to focus its efforts through the TCU group. The DFWHC has continued to support the TCU Collaborative in several ways, including distribution of Collaborative meeting notices, offers to attend Web-based conferences, and making Collaborative members aware of joint hospital data already being collected by the DFWHC Data Initiative. Through this sharing, Collaborative members learned that extensive joint data, of which many members were unaware, already is available to members of the TCU Collaborative.

HOSPITAL PERSPECTIVE

Chief nurse executives, Magnet project directors, and nurse researchers in Magnet-designated organizations and those on the "Journey to Excellence" feel both a responsibility for and a commitment to evidence-based practice, nursing research, and community partnerships with local colleges of nursing. One of the difficulties in this particular urban area is that relationships between academia and service do not exist within systems and must be facilitated, implemented, and sustained by forging partnerships between nurse leaders in university and health care system settings to share scarce faculty resources across settings and accomplish mutual goals.

As members of the TCU EBPR Collaborative, the perspective of area hospitals is that the Collaborative serves as an excellent vehicle for networking with other nurse leaders who share common vision and purpose. The Collaborative offers the possibility of working together to create training programs in evidence-based practice and research and to collaborate on multisite clinical studies while efficiently capitalizing on the wealth of nursing talent in a large, diverse metropolitan area. Despite the competitive nature of this environment, nurses can come together around the table to share both unique and similar perspectives regarding the issues that affect both patients and nurses. This Collaborative provides a forum for brainstorming ideas and sharing best practices and eventually may make possible the implementation of multisite projects with greater scientific rigor than could be accomplished by any one of these organizations acting alone.

One of the difficulties in contracting with a single entity or individual for nursing research consultation is that the organization may be limited by the specific clinical expertise and research experience of a single individual and academic setting. With the rich diversity of nurse researchers, expert clinicians, and organizations within the Collaborative, the members are connected efficiently to a broader environment of resources and possibilities for partnerships.

In light of limited internal and external funding and organizational resources, this initiative connects nursing experts in efficient ways to assist members in identifying evidence-based best practices that result in quality patient outcomes and therefore provides a beneficial solution for all involved. A single entity or individual cannot provide sufficient infrastructure to support the same level of evidence-based practice and research education and consultation that is possible through a large collaborative effort such as that offered by the TCU EBPR Collaborative. Individuals responsible for evidence-based practice and research programs in area organizations feel fortunate to be part of an initiative of this magnitude that brings nurse leaders, clinicians, and researchers together to foster scientific inquiry, educate direct-care nurses about evidence-based practice and research, and create safe environments for patients.

SUCCESSES

The activities of the TCU EBPR Collaborative have resulted in many benefits. TCU has enjoyed a long-standing positive relationship with numerous clinical agencies, and those relationships have been strengthened even further through the Collaborative. The Collaborative is a tangible demonstration of the university's commitment to improving nursing practice and patient care in area hospitals. This commitment has been reciprocated by the hospitals' support of the Collaborative and their use of TCU nursing faculty members as consultants for EBPR projects. Another benefit has been a strengthened relationship between nursing faculty members from three different universities who are providing EBPR consultation services to various hospitals. The joint pool of talent among these faculty members, as well as among the nurse researchers employed by area hospitals, is significant and provides a wealth of opportunity for joint support and projects. Hospitals that are on the Magnet journey have been mentored by other hospitals that are already Magnet-designated, and hospitals with current Magnet designation have received encouragement and ideas from their peer agencies.

An encouraging milestone occurred during the third meeting of the TCU EBPR Collaborative when a poster that had been presented at a recent national nursing conference was discussed. The poster described a similar collaborative that had developed among Magnet-designated hospitals in a much larger urban setting. In comparison, the TCU Collaborative developed quickly over a 6-month period with significantly more hospitals as members. Another unique feature of the TCU Collaborative was the inclusion of faculty members from three universities, as well as the actual sponsorship of the Collaborative by the primary university.

FUTURE GOALS

The future goals of the TCU EBPR Collaborative are categorized in three primary realms: continued sharing of best practices, development of an EBP Fellowship for direct-care nurses, and joint benchmarking and research. The EBP Fellowship planning is progressing, and it is anticipated that the Fellowship will begin in the fall of 2008. TCU faculty members and nurse researchers from area hospitals have offered to serve as the faculty and facilitators of the Fellowship. Support such as facilities, continuing education credit, and other supplies will be requested from hospitals whose direct-care nurses participate in the EBP Fellowship. In addition, there will be a fee for each participating nurse to cover the additional costs of the Fellowship.

A goal that is not as well defined at this point is the joint benchmarking and research. An area of interest is joint research about nurse-sensitive indicators and the possible opportunity to benchmark at the regional level. The DFWHC Data Initiative has offered to provide opportunities for shared data, and additional projects probably will develop. One idea being considered is a research project regarding the relationship of nurse-sensitive indicators to nursing turnover and vacancy.

The meetings of the TCU EBPR Collaborative have been highly valued as forums for sharing, brainstorming, and problem solving. It is anticipated that this type of collegial exchange will remain one of the most valued aspects of the Collaborative. In addition, the hosting of speakers who are recognized experts from outside the Dallas-Fort Worth area is seen as an area of focus for future events.

SUMMARY

As health care has become increasingly more complex, the tendency is to engage in detailed strategic planning, constantly refine processes, and attempt to control closely all aspects of practice. The TCU EBPR Collaborative has been a successful example of an initiative that began in simple brainstorming, was allowed to evolve, and gradually developed into a highly valued endeavor. The initial concern about the attempt to foster collaboration among competitors has not proved to be an issue. During the initial meeting of the Collaborative, one CNO in attendance responded to the concern about competition by stating that the Collaborative could be successful if it focused on doing what was right for patients and what was right for nurses. With those priorities in mind, any concerns about competition have been resolved quickly. The Collaborative holds great potential for significantly affecting patient safety and quality of care on a regional level.

Renewing the Spirit of Nursing: Embracing Evidence-Based Practice in a Rural State

Ann E. Sossong, RN, PhD[a],*, Sue Cullen, RN, MSN[b],
Paula Theriault, RN, MBA[c], Alanna Stetson, RN, BSN, BC[d],
Barbara Higgins, RNC, PhD[e], Sarina Roche, RNC, DNSc[f],
Sue Ellis-Hermansen, RN, MS[g], Dorrin Patillo, RN-B[h]

KEYWORDS

- Evidence-based practice • Quality care
- Collaborative partnerships • Consortium
- Barriers • Rural state

The nursing profession has been challenged to develop and implement improved patient care outcomes that are supported by research findings. These efforts are supported by the Institute of Medicine's (IOM) report that identifies a health care safety crisis, citing an increase in preventable deaths in the United States.[1,2] The IOM (2001) report clearly calls for nursing and other health care disciplines to care for patients using best evidence and encourages professionals to move practice more quickly to the application of research findings in the clinical setting.[3,4] The IOM report highlights the need to restructure health care delivery to create systems that are both patient centered and evidence based.[3] Organizations in which health care takes place must be dynamic and adaptive to appropriate internal and external feedback based on

[a] School of Nursing, 5765 Dunn Hall, University of Maine, Orono, ME 04469, USA
[b] Education Department, Acadia Hospital, 268 Stillwater Avenue, Bangor, ME 04401, USA
[c] Education Department, St. Joseph Hospital, 360 Broadway, Bangor, ME 04401, USA
[d] Education and Training Center, Eastern Maine Medical Center, Eastern Maine Healthcare, Whiting Hill, Brewer, ME 04412, USA
[e] Department of Nursing, Husson College, One College Circle, Bangor, ME 04401, USA
[f] Department of Nursing, Eastern Maine Community College, 354 Hogan Road, Bangor, ME 04401, USA
[g] Omicron Xi Chapter At-Large, Sigma Theta Tau International Honor Society, School of Nursing, 5765 Dunn Hall, University of Maine, Orono, ME 04469, USA
[h] Education Department, Dorothea Dix Psychiatric Center, 656 State Street, Bangor, ME 04401, USA
* Corresponding author.
E-mail address: ann.sossong@umit.maine.edu (A.E. Sossong).

Nurs Clin N Am 44 (2009) 33–42
doi:10.1016/j.cnur.2008.10.010
0029-6465/08/$ – see front matter © 2009 Elsevier Inc. All rights reserved.

nursing.theclinics.com

evidence but structured enough to maintain order in a complex and ever-changing system.

When a complex institutional system is organized purposefully to be dynamic, clinical practice is transformed more easily to ensure patient safety and quality of care. Such systems contain mechanisms for continual feedback on selected outcomes, as well as regular and frequent searches for solutions to problems that have been identified. Evidence-based practice (EBP) is an essential part of the strategy used to accomplish this positive transformation. As Melnyk and Fineout-Overholt[5] purport, "EBP is a problem-solving approach to practice, one that cultivates an excitement for implementing the highest quality care as well as a spirit of inquiry and life-long learning." Acknowledging the role of EBP is an essential step in achieving quality outcomes.

An informal interdisciplinary group of educational leaders began to meet at the University of Maine in 2006 to undertake a dialogue about how to accomplish a transformation to EBP that ensures patient safety and improved quality of care. Members of the group represented the nursing honor society, acute and critical access hospitals, mental health institutions, and university and college schools of nursing in central and northern regions of Maine. Collaborative efforts to introduce and implement EBP in these areas in Maine were deliberate and focused, although initially there was no clear vision of the outcome.

This article provides insight into the formative processes of the group, discusses the collaborative efforts of the group, and describes the outcomes. The IOM challenge to implement EBP is addressed as a central theme, and a process has been established that continually revisits the quality of that transformational implementation, even in the more remote areas of Maine.

THE JOURNEY BEGINS

Nursing leaders must form strong informal and formal networks in any geographic area if high standards of care are to be met and maintained. It could be argued that successful and effective links in these networks are more important in a large rural state like Maine than in more densely populated ares of the country. Frequent interactions between educators and health care institutions are necessary simply because of the need for agreements regarding clinical articulation and professional development programs within and among representative organizations. Discussions during these interactions revealed a common desire to integrate EBP in health care organizations and academia, but no one had a clear idea how to accomplish this goal. The shared value of incorporating EBP into agency or institutional policies helped the group stay focused and led to discussion about the need to change nursing culture to reflect this value. Central to the conversation was the need to clarify challenges and barriers to change from each participant's perspective.

All members of the interdisciplinary group previously had attended a program in which Alyce Schultz,[6] RN, PhD, had spoken about a successful Clinical Scholar Model (CSM) and mentorship program for EBP in the southeastern (more urban) part of Maine. Dr. Schultz's earlier presentations had familiarized the group with examples of clinical scholarship initiatives. The group also was familiar with other clinical scholar models, such as the ACE Star Model of evidence-based nursing practice,[7] the Stetler model of research use to promote EBP,[8] and the Iowa Model of EBP to promote quality.[9] Each of the models emphasize "clinical scholarship as an intellectual process, steeped in curiosity that challenges traditional nursing practice through observation, analysis, synthesis, application, and dissemination."[7] The success of earlier educational programs in southeastern Maine was attributed to the use of the CSM along with teamwork and collaboration. The nursing leaders realized this same team-work and collaborative spirit had to be essential elements in the process, regardless of locale, if they were to engage the nurses in EBP.[10,11]

Another element in creating and maintaining a culture of clinical excellence re-quired more attention to additional collaborative partnerships with major stake-holders (eg, leadership from tertiary health care centers and critical access hospitals). Partnerships between nursing and these institutional representatives fo-cusing on improvements in patient care afford educational leaders more opportuni-ties to design educational programs that facilitate the integration of shared values of EBP. These steps are a logical part of the process for cultivating professional pride and excitement.[6] Through these collaborative efforts, educational leaders are able to establish a more deliberate and organized approach for creating a culture of change by gaining the support of key organizational leaders in cultivating a spirit of inquiry. The value placed on inquiry (versus tradition or simple habit) will lead nurses to acquire a better knowledge base for practice, which is a necessary step to inform and facilitate better patient outcomes.

PAVING THE WAY

As in any endeavor of this magnitude, barriers surfaced that required patience and perseverance to overcome. Some of these obstacles were expected, and others were encountered during the team-building process. Those in more rural areas were relatively unfamiliar with the meaning of EBP. Some of the nurses in the group identified lack of time to explore and adopt protocols reflecting EBP as a barrier to change. Other nurses who were fully engaged in research projects did not recognize the ways in which their findings were applicable and were hesitant to share results with colleagues. These experiences were consistent with the findings of Nagy and colleagues,[12] who found four major obstacles to the use of EBP in their study of nurse's beliefs about the conditions that hinder or support evidence-based nursing. These major obstacles include "nurses' lack of belief in the use of evidence to guide practice, lack of organizational support, lack of time to use evidence effectively in practice, and lack of knowledge in the use of evidence."[12]

Competitive tension also existed between various organizational and educational leaders. Nursing initiatives in the different settings customarily were developed without input from others, and this pattern did not foster collaborative thinking or efforts. Introspection during the group meetings led to the realization that such ini-tiatives had been seen as responses to internal conditions of the institution rather than processes that better might be seen as reactions to broader national or state-wide events. Long-standing rivalries and a history of actions directed at local-only interests led to ineffective support for collaborative efforts between administration in health care and academic settings. As honest dialogue progressed, the goal of creating a clinical scholar environment for nursing emerged. The group energy that resulted from this positive dynamic was certainly a factor that fed the change process.

It is necessary to inform organizational leaders of the importance of EBP as part of the process of reinforcing the changes needed in institutional culture. Literature on systems change emphasizes the need to avoid the roadblocks and pitfalls that often hinder staff-driven initiatives and to promote organizational champions. Even though sustaining EBP is a difficult task, the difficulty does not detract from the value of the endeavor.[13] Champions of this cultural change surface through strategic initiatives to provide optimal outcomes for patients, thereby creating a culture of excellence.

THE PROCESS OF SOLIDIFYING A COLLABORATIVE PARTNERSHIP

The first step in establishing this partnership was to acknowledge the underlying competitive tension between the various organizations. The shared value for evidence-based nursing practice gave participants a common connection from which to build the trust needed to conduct this dialogue. Members in the group agreed that Dr. Schultz would be ideally suited to guide the task ahead. She was familiar with the culture, challenges, and historical relationships between and among institutions represented in the group. Her credibility as an expert in successfully establishing a CSM allowed members of the group to welcome her guidance.[14]

The CSM is a logical process of implementing research and therefore sustaining the use of evidence in nursing practice. This model requires strategies for organizational support and teamwork.[14] Dr. Schultz's previous success in implementing the CSM with the assistance of several point-of-care nurse researchers was recognized nationally and internationally. her enthusiasm and familiarity with the process instilled a belief that the initiative to cultivate and institute EBP was not only desirable but also was attainable.

Meetings were held in which Dr. Schultz and other southern Maine colleagues graciously shared their experiences with the CSM. These brainstorming sessions led to the decision to hold an inquiry-based learning workshop as a necessary means of institutionalizing EBP. All participants needed greater familiarity with the notion of both doing and teaching EBP; that familiarity in turn would reinforce the connections that were necessary for successful long-term change. The workshop would help the group develop a common language for educational goals that would be appropriate for nurses and administrators. Sessions within the workshop needed to provide opportunities for nurses to gain an understanding of what EBP was (and was not) and to evaluate and appraise critically the quality of research findings. Likewise, workshop sessions were needed to provide administrators with guidance on how to support EBP institutionally and ultimately infuse research findings into the practice environment by using an EBP model.

The agencies to which individual members of the group belonged were asked for contributions to cover the expense involved in the workshop. There was support from representative organizations for the workshop, although resources were limited. Dr. Schultz generously donated her time and expertise to the endeavor, and the seeds for creating a comprehensive event to cultivate EBP in rural Maine were planted.

THE WORKSHOP: PROMOTING EVIDENCE-BASED PRACTICE THROUGH A SPIRIT OF INQUIRY: 2007

The theme of the 1-day workshop promoting EBP through a spirit of inquiry. The educational leaders in the group worked closely with Dr. Schultz, who then was the Associate Director for the Advancement of Evidence-Based Practice at Arizona State University, College of Nursing and Health care Innovation. In the spring of 2007 the well-attended workshop was held in central Maine, a location that was reasonably accessible to the target audience. Participants came from many of the state's rural health care organizations. Most of the conference attendees were staff nurses, although several organizations were represented by administrators.

An introductory session in the workshop addressed the dynamics of managing change, with attention to the feasibility and sustainability of EBP. An element in this portion of the workshop was the need to identify the characteristics of a transformational leader—a role model who leads nurses to question practice and rewards changes and innovation. These mentors "walk the talk" by continually asking for the evidence, strengthening their knowledge and skills related to reading and appraising research, and demonstrating willingness to change practice if evidence contradicts beliefs.[15] Another early task was to address the need for innovative leaders who could create an infrastructure to support EBP. The interactive workshop allowed participants to explore their values in relation to the characteristics of a transformational leader and to identify strategies for change within their own institution's culture.

The structured sessions in the workshop included collaborative exercises designed to stimulate ideas for research projects among the participants. Examples of studies focusing on the patient/nurse interface at the point of care were used to assist participants in conceptualizing clinical issues. Participants also were assisted in easily identifying sources for existing evidence and methods for evaluating the quality of that evidence. A medical librarian was an invaluable resource for this part of the workshop. The librarian provided detailed and specific information about how to locate and select the best refereed research articles supporting EBP and how to locate and evaluate clinical practice guidelines. The importance of addressing the use and implementation of these guidelines in nursing practice was considered separately, with time allowed for specific questions that might arise at a particular institution. Workshop participants were introduced to the essential requirements and strategies for implementing EBP and to barriers to implementation previously identified in the literature.[9]

Another feature in the workshop was the "Evidence in Action" panel. This discussion panel included expert nurses, a director of clinical research, and a physician at a large tertiary center in central Maine. The "spirit of inquiry" theme was reinforced by the panel participants reminding attendees that many institutional protocols had been developed by nurses as they tried to improve patient care. Panelists and attendees acknowledged that there had been an ongoing, although less formal, level of nursing research supporting EBP in their organizations that affected quality improvement processes. Participants saw that change was possible and that the mechanisms for such change already were partially in place. The major learning objective for the workshop was to recognize the value of incorporating research findings into practice guidelines that would result in improvements in clinical outcomes. Workshop attendees also were expected to communicate their readiness to implement EBP in their respective work settings.

THE MAINE NURSING PRACTICE CONSORTIUM

Nursing leaders debriefed after the EBP workshop expressed the need to establish a more permanent collaborative group, resulting in the formation of the Maine Nursing Practice Consortium (MNPC). The MNPC has evolved and continues to be a valuable resource helping bridge the cultural differences between research-rich urban health science centers and the smaller medical centers and critical access hospitals that constitute the more rural Maine health care systems. Following the first workshop, the MNPC members worked diligently with nurses in their respective institutions to promote EBP. They met regularly to share the progress of EBP initiatives, and more formal arrangements were made between and within institutions to implement EBP. Members were committed to promoting the goals of the partnership and to working to maintain the momentum for the spirit of inquiry. Professional pride in accomplishments was evident among those who played a part in the first workshop, and a sense of shared achievement provided a base from which to set clear goals for continued evidence-based efforts of the MNPC.

Shared values among MNPC members had to be agreed upon before collegial relationships could be established between the nurse educators and the health care providers and administrators of the health care systems. In most cases, increased and improved communication between the nursing leaders was a necessary step in incorporating EBP into regular dialogue among nurse educators, nurses at the bedside, and administrators in institutional settings where health care is provided. Educational workshops as well as collaborative partnerships such as the MNPC were essential to advance nursing in the quest for optimal patient care outcomes.

FIRST YEAR ACCOMPLISHMENTS

Organizational commitment to the collaborative efforts was stronger after the workshop, as measured by offers of time and financial support for the mission of instituting EBP. Nurses who attended the conference began searching literature pertinent to their nursing projects, no doubt aided by the knowledge shared at the conference. Nursing leaders who participated in the workshop development worked more collaboratively, using teamwork to advance the goals of safety and quality patient care. A shared appreciation of the value of EBP, continually reinforcing the language and processes aimed at a spirit of inquiry, was leading inevitably to outcomes recommended by professional, accrediting, and regulatory organizations at all levels.

More collaborative avenues developed as a direct result of increased organizational understanding of the components of EBP. Experiential opportunities for senior nursing students were initiated, providing them with beginning skills and knowledge in the research process and use of evidence that they can incorporate into their own EBP. A Nursing Research Fellowship is being sought for graduate nursing students.

There is lively dialogue at area hospitals aimed at identifying ways in which staff can implement EBP routinely on the various clinical units. One study, "Patients' and Nurses' Perceptions of Caring," recently completed by academic faculty and staff nurses, represents the first successful research collaboration. The impetus for the study was the increased emphasis hospitals place on marketing their institutions as the best place to come for care. What constitutes excellent care is difficult to define, especially from the patient's perspective. To implement true patient-centered care, it is essential to incorporate the patient perspective on caring. This study provided evidence about what both patients and nurses perceived as "care." Findings from this collaborative study have been presented nationally and internationally and have been well received. The process provided the leadership of the hospital with the chance to acknowledge the significance of nursing contributions in improving patient satisfaction and quality of care. This study was the first independent nursing study conducted at this central Maine hospital, because nursing studies previously had required physician sponsorship. When the proposal for this study was submitted to the institutional review board for approval, the clinical research director worked with academic faculty to change the policy to allow nurses to engage in research that promotes EBP without physician sponsorship.

Another successful outcome of these collaborative activities is visible at the world's only psychiatric hospital with Magnet designation. This psychiatric and substance abuse facility in central Maine now formally and institutionally embraces nursing practices that are evidence based. The facility's chief nursing officer attended the 2007 workshop and strongly supported the spirit of inquiry. This Magnet hospital uses nursing leadership teams to infuse the principles of EBP through research. The concept has permeated the institution and includes advanced-practice registered nurses and staff nurses in the collaborative process.

The educational workshop sessions promoted a change in the perception of what constitutes research, identified research activities as "doable" by nurses, and incorporated the value of practice based on evidence for all who attended. Perhaps the most fundamental outcome is the recognition that EBP is part of the professional role of all nurses, whether they are brainstorming about what research is needed, searching for supporting evidence to inform a particular practice, writing a proposal, or gathering data as part of a clinical project. Examples of evidence-based projects inspired by the 2007 workshop are varied (eg, constipation-relieving remedies for patients on methadone therapy, intravenous fluid hydration for postprocedure electroconvulsive therapy for patients suffering from headaches, and nurses and EBP in a successful school re-entry project), but all represent the movement toward a "spirit of inquiry."

The successful outcomes from the workshop have contributed immeasurably to a change in the perception of the role of nurses as researchers and change agents for EBP in their respective institutions. There is greater confidence in nurses' ability and greater institutional support for the establishment of an environment for research leading to evidence-driven practice. Clearly, there has been a shift from lip service about the value of EBP to acknowledgment of the responsibility of all nurses at all levels for creating a favorable institutional setting in which nurses implement EBP. Change in systems and practice stimulated by the workshop sessions has been brought to bear in this geographically large but rural environment. Success from the initial workshop led to the development of the second EBP workshop in April 2008.

RENEWING THE SPIRIT OF NURSING: 2008

Sensing a renewed spirit, the MNPC members designed the second EBP workshop to provide novice nurses the opportunity to speak about and showcase their work. Workshop organizers believed that the focus on accomplishments would convey effectively the value placed on EBP. The recognition of achievements energized and encouraged nurses to continue to direct their energy toward systematic evaluation and promotion of EBP. Nurse researchers well versed in the use of EBP strategies who had presented in the 2007 workshop returned to evaluate and recognize achievements and build more clear connections between EBP and a higher quality of patient care.

Jane Kirschling, RN, DNS, Dean and Professor of University of Kentucky, College of Nursing, and former Dean at the University of Southern Maine, provided the keynote address at "Renewing the Spirit of Nursing by Embracing EBP 2008." She reinforced the call for EBP and emphasized the implications of national initiatives on nursing practice. Expanding on the previous workshop initiatives, she helped the participants identify their expanded roles, influence, and responsibility to assure that nursing practice is examined critically and is assessed systematically to provide quality care. Interactive sessions enabled the nurses to gain further insight in how the national initiatives from organizations such as the Agency for Health Care Research and Quality, National Quality Forum, National Database of Nursing Quality Indicators, and Quality and Safety in Nursing Education affect decisions made by leaders in changing health care systems in their institutions.

The language of these initiatives encompassed EBP to generate measurable, optimal patient outcomes. The participants acknowledged that they shared a common change, because all the national nursing initiatives mirrored their efforts to promote optimal patient care by changing systems and practices, with the ultimate goal of ensuring

Box 1
Selected EBP projects presented at "Renewing the Spirit of Nursing: 2008"

Implementation of sucrose for neonatal procedural pain

Nursing role: nonpharmacologic interventions for insomnia

Providing behavioral health care in primary practice settings: co-location pilot project

Inflammatory bowel disease in children: an overview for the pediatric health care provider

Health Lifestyles Group: nursing practice improves patient outcomes

Therapeutic hypothermia following out-of-hospital cardiac arrest

Psychiatric emergency response team outcomes

safety and improving quality outcomes through best evidence. These national initiatives have opened doors previously closed to nursing, and the participants recognized that there are greater opportunities for nurses to assume a leadership role in a dynamic, challenging, and increasingly complex health care system.

OUTCOMES OF THE 2007 AND 2008 WORKSHOPS

Advances in EBP in central and northern Maine as a result the 2007 and 2008 workshops are evident when considering the quality and the quantity of projects presented by staff nurses in 2008 (**Box 1**). Positive outcomes in the "Renewing the Spirit of Nursing 2008" workshop were evident in the outcomes of the projects presented by nurses and in staff nurses' active participation. Enthusiasm for the change was expressed through verbal and written communications and evaluations that demonstrated increased knowledge regarding EBP, greater familiarity with national initiatives concerning EBP, and individual contributions to organizational changes.

LESSONS LEARNED

MNPC members have categorized their experiences into six major lessons for the development of EBP in rural Maine. These insights may prove useful to other groups of leaders who are committed to a similar vision for promoting collaborative efforts among academic institutions and health care systems in rural settings.

1. Communication among nurses in clinal practice, nurse educators, and those in administrative positions is essential for the creation of a dialogue for change in the culture of nursing. Collaboration is based on effective communication.
2. Clear professional nursing goals can supersede individual organizational goals when competing factions in nursing can overcome rivalry.
3. Logistic challenges to meetings for participants in wide geographic areas can be overcome when all members commit to participation in a manner that acknowledges individual circumstances.
4. When the ultimate goal is to provide the safest and highest-quality nursing care to the citizens in rural areas, funds and material resources will not be a prohibitive factor to progress.
5. Patience and respect for colleagues are essential qualities for a collaborative team process, regardless of the goal.
6. The driver for change must be the common goal of patient safety and quality care, not individual or institutional advantage.

SUMMARY

A group of nursing leaders from several organizations in the central and northern regions of the state established the MNPC. Their efforts renewed the spirit of nursing through a commitment to collaborate on the adoption and integration of EBP in each clinical and educational setting. Regular meetings with this goal in mind led to the design of workshops focusing on the establishment and continued promotion of EBP. Trust was established within and between organizations, geographic and traditionally competitive barriers were addressed, and members of the MNPC led a number of evidence-based initiatives.

Staff nurses acknowledged the value of their evidence-based unit improvement projects and proudly showcased these results. Faculty members in schools of nursing continue to pursue better methods for integrating EBP in undergraduate and graduate nursing courses. Faculty members also incorporate national initiatives into classroom discussions as well as clinical practice settings. Nursing administrators likewise are embracing EBP and strongly support nurses in their quest to improve patient care by revising practices through mechanisms based on the best evidence.

Renewing the spirit of nursing through EBP was a challenge that was met in central and northern Maine through the collaborative efforts of committed nursing leaders. The consortium members created a synergy for valuing, using, teaching, and adding to the professionalism of nursing through EBP. The incorporation of EBP as a fundamental concept in nursing practice was given a tremendous boost with a modest beginning of respectful dialogue that has led rural Maine nurses in academia and practice institutions to excel. Members of the MNPC will continue to foster collaborative efforts that support and strengthen EBP endeavors in rural Maine. Excellence in clinical care and improvement of patient outcomes result from applying the intellectual process in the application of new scientific knowledge. There is reason to believe that EBP also can become a reality in the even more rural areas of Maine, and this goal is more likely to be realized if team spirit and collaborative effort play a key part In the process.

ACKNOWLEDGMENT

The authors acknowledge Carol Wood, EdD, Graduate Coordinator, School of Nursing, University of Maine, Orono, ME, for her editing and support.

REFERENCES

1. Kohn LT, Corrigan JM, Donaldson MS, editors. To err is human: building a safer health system. Washington, DC: National Academy Press; 2000.
2. Aspden P, Corrigan JM, Wolcott J, editors. Patient safety: achieving a new standard for care. Washington, DC: The National Academies Press; 2004.
3. Committee on the Quality of Health Care in America. Crossing the quality chasm: a new health system for the 21st century. Washington, DC: National Academy Press; 2001.
4. Finkelman A, Kenner C. Teaching IOM: implications of the Institute of Medicine reports for nursing education. Silver Spring (MD): American Nurses Association; 2007.
5. Melnyk BM, Fineout-Overholt E. Evidence-based practice in nursing & healthcare: a guide to best practice. Philadelphia: Lippincott Williams & Wilkins; 2005.

6. Schultz AA. Origins and aspirations: conceiving the Clinical Scholar Model. Excellence in Nursing Knowledge 2005;6:1–4. Available at: http://www.nursingknowledge.org/Portal/Main.aspx?PageId=3512&IssueNo=6. Accessed May 17, 2008.

7. Stevens KR. ACE Star Model of EBP: knowledge transformation. Academic Center for Evidence-based Practice, The University of Texas Health Science Center at San Antonia; 2004. Available at: www.acestar.uthscsa.edu. Accessed June 19, 2008.

8. Stetler CB. Updating the Stetler model of research utilization to facilitate evidence-based practice. Nurs Outlook 2001;49(6):272–9.

9. Titler MG, Kleiber C, Steelman VJ, et al. The Iowa model of evidence-based practice to promote quality care. Crit Care Nurs Clin North Am 2001;13(4):497–509. Available at: http://www.ncbi.nlm.nih.gov/pubmed/11778337. Accessed May 17, 2008.

10. Schultz AA. Implementation: a team effort. Nurs Manage 2007;38(6):12–4. Available at: http://www.nursingcenter.com/Library/JournalArticle.asp?Article_ID=718987. Accessed May 17, 2008.

11. Schultz AA. The Clinical Scholar Model: promoting interdisciplinary EBP teamwork at the point of care. Presented at the 18th International Nursing Research Congress Focusing on EBP. Vienna, Austria, July 12, 2007. Available at: http://stti.confex.com/stti/congrs07/techprogram/paper_33398.htm. Accessed May 17, 2008.

12. Nagy S, Lumby J, McKinley S, et al. Nurses' belief about the conditions that hinder or support evidence-based nursing. Int J Nurs Pract 2001;7:314–21.

13. Stetler CB, Caramanica L. Evaluation of an evidence-based practice initiative: outcomes, strengths and limitations of a retrospective, conceptually-based approach. Blackwell Synergy-Worldviews Evid Based Nurs 2007;4(4):187–99.

14. Schultz AA. Clinical scholars at the bedside: an EBP mentorship model for today. Excellence in Nursing Knowledge 2005;6:1–8. Available at: http://www.nursingknowledge.org/Portal/Main.aspx?PageId=3512&IssueNo=6. Accessed May 17, 2008.

15. Schultz AA. Sustainability of EBP: learning organizations. Presented at Promoting Evidence Based-practice Through a Spirit of Inquiry. Eastern Maine Community College, Bangor (ME), April 6, 2007.

Implementing a Health System-Wide Evidence-Based Practice Educational Program to Reach Nurses with Various Levels of Experience and Educational Preparation

Teri Britt Pipe, PhD, RN[a],*, Jane A. Timm, MS, RN[b],
Marcelline R. Harris, PhD, RN[c], Doreen K. Frusti, MSN, MS, RN[b],
Sharon Tucker, PhD, RN[b], Jaqueline M. Attlesey-Pries, MS, RN[d],
Katherine Brady-Schluttner, MS, RN-BC[e], Julie Neumann, MS, RN[e],
J. Wayne Street, RN[f], Diane Twedell, DNP, RN[e], Marianne Olson, PhD, RN[b],
Gina Long, DNSc, RN[a], Cindy Scherb, PhD, RN[b]

KEYWORDS

- Evidence-based practice • Leadership
- Nursing professional development • Practice innovation
- Informatics • National Quality Forum

The NQF Scholars Program was funded by the Mayo Clinic Rochester Board through the Incented Investment in Mayo's Future.

[a] Nursing Research, Division of Nursing, Mayo Clinic College of Medicine, Mayo Clinic Arizona, Mayo Clinic Hospital, Nursing Administration, 5777 E. Mayo Boulevard, Phoenix, AZ 85054, USA
[b] Nursing Research Division, Department of Nursing, Mayo Clinic College of Medicine, Mayo Clinic Rochester, 200 SW 1st Street, Rochester, MN 55905, USA
[c] Division of Nursing Informatics and Nursing Health Sciences Research, Department of Nursing, Mayo Clinic Rochester, 200 SW 1st Street, Rochester, MN 55905, USA
[d] Nursing Practice Resource Division, Department of Nursing, Mayo Clinic Rochester, 200 SW 1st Street, Rochester, MN 55905, USA
[e] Education and Professional Development Division, Department of Nursing, Mayo Clinic Rochester, 200 SW 1st Street, Rochester, MN 55905, USA
[f] Nursing Trauma, Luther Midelfort, 1221 Whipple Street, Eau Claire, WI 54701, USA
* Corresponding author.
E-mail address: pipe.teri@mayo.edu (T.B. Pipe).

Nurs Clin N Am 44 (2009) 43–55
doi:10.1016/j.cnur.2008.10.008
0029-6465/08/$ – see front matter © 2009 Elsevier Inc. All rights reserved.

nursing.theclinics.com

The work of nursing always has changed with the times, remaining rooted in theoretic and ethical foundations but being flexible enough to expand and meet new challenges. The emerging and future work of nursing requires a growing agility to allow the practitioner to move between disparate knowledge areas and to integrate cognitive skill sets in creative and innovative ways. Three of these areas of knowledge are clinical informatics, evidence-based practice (EBP), and nursing-sensitive quality methodologies. Until recently these content domains have been absent from the academic and service education curricula. When content has been provided, these three domains have been learned and applied separately. In the evolving health care arena, it became apparent to Mayo Clinic Nursing that preparing nurses with expertise in all of these content areas would position the health care system to deliver the best scientifically grounded care for patients and to communicate clinical information and outcomes of care effectively for the mutual benefits of the patient, nurse, and the organization. Thus, the departments and divisions of nursing embarked on a system-wide educational initiative to expand the knowledge of nursing leaders in clinical informatics, EBP, and nursing-sensitive quality methodologies as well as the skills needed to translate this knowledge into optimal impact at the point of patient care. Intramural funding was secured to develop, execute, and evaluate the initiative.

The system designed and implemented a 1-year curriculum for nurses that focused on the three content domains of clinical informatics, EBP, and quality methodologies. This article describes a system-wide EBP educational initiative implemented with a geographically, educationally, and clinically diverse group of direct care nurses with the intent of increasing their EBP skill set and their efficacy as local change agents and leaders. In this article, the overall program is described, and then the focus is narrowed to describe the EBP components of the initiative with case examples and lessons learned. Although the National Quality Forum (NQF) Scholars Program was much broader in scope, only the EBP components of the program are presented as examples.

NATIONAL QUALITY FORUM SCHOLARS INITIATIVE

The initiative was named the "NQF Scholars Program." This name was selected to denote the rigorous academic preparation combined with the context of nursing-sensitive quality indicators published by the National Quality Forum.[1] The vision was to expand the knowledge of nursing leaders to translate best practices into optimal impact at the direct point of patient care through focusing on the NQF nursing-sensitive measure set.[1] The result envisioned was enhanced effectiveness in nursing practice by decreases in unnecessary variation across all of the systems' health care facilities guided by a shared mission of doing what is best for the patient.

The approach described in this article is a departure from the local hospital–based efforts that have been presented elsewhere.[2–8] In the past, the efforts designed to improve EBP knowledge and skills were directed primarily at the local organizational level; this initiative provided the opportunity to broaden the scope and coordination of efforts to a system-wide perspective that encompassed nursing professionals across Mayo Clinic's five-state health care enterprise, including the affiliated multistate health care system. The essence of this program was to create and apply rigorous academic preparation with the primary focus on patient quality and safety from a nursing perspective.

The model guiding the EBP portion of the curriculum was the Clinical Scholar Model.[9] The Clinical Scholar Model promotes a spirit of inquiry and willingness to change the processes and tasks of patient care and the theories framing practice based on rigorous, systematic appraisal of the evidence guided by nursing clinical judgement. The approach is one of mentorship that supports nurses in becoming responsible, account-able change agents for providing patient care based on the best evidence available.[9]

NQF SCHOLARS: A PROGRAM DESCRIPTION

Numerous organizations, including the Institute of Medicine, the NQF, and the Joint Commission on Accreditation of Healthcare Organizations, have recognized that EBP, performance measurement sets, and health information technologies are critical to improving the quality and safety of health care. The current program was developed and implemented to prepare registered nurses to be NQF scholars by combining curriculum from each of these concepts (**Table 1** provides a curriculum overview and prototypical schedule). This program was designed to establish a critical foundation for the future of nursing across the Mayo Health System by addressing the five core competencies recommended by the Institute of Medicine, which also include key factors that are known to affect directly the recruitment and retention of nurses:[10]

- Demonstration of the highest quality of care using nursing-sensitive outcome measures
- Demonstration of organizational support for ongoing learning and EBP
- Practicing nurse involvement in key processes
- Exposure to the research foundations for practice
- Access to and use of information technologies in the workplace

Table 1
Nursing National Quality Forum Scholar Program: schedule at a glance

Dates	Activity	Location
Month 1	Quality Conference Networking event "Sustaining the Gains" for Cohort 1 Scholars "Setting the Stage for NQF Scholars" for Cohort 2 Scholars	Central site
Months 2–4	Informatics AMIA 10 × 10 online course	Local setting
Months 5–6	Informatics synthesis Networking event Evidence-based practice overview	Central site
Months 6–7	Summer assignment: information gathering at local setting about related initiatives and contacts	Local setting
Month 8	Evidence-based practice kick-off System-wide quality model Data governance presentation Evening networking event	Central site
Months 8–11	Online evidence-based practice course via virtual classroom (12 modules) Statistical concepts Translating course concepts into National Quality Forum project/project development	Local setting
Months 11–12	Virtual meeting for project presentations and National Quality Forum leadership role Project implementation	Local setting
Month 12	Nursing Research Conference Evening recognition/social event	Central site

SPECIFIC PROGRAM GOALS

The specific aims of the NQF Scholars Program were to prepare practicing nurse scholars to

1. Serve as local leaders and champions of nursing-focused and/or nursing-relevant NQF measure sets and their associated EBP
2. Use Web-based tools on the system-wide intranet for collecting evidence, conducting analysis, sharing information, and benchmarking
3. Bring forward and apply informatics principles at their sites

The program development team consisted of the chief nurse executive with oversight of the entire organizational system, faculty members with expertise in the three content domains, and administrative project planners whose role it was to coordinate the efforts of the entire team and manage the logistics of the program from enrollment to evaluation. A steering group consisting of members of the program development team and other key nursing leaders guided the initiative in a strategic and effective direction. Members of the faculty and the administrative project planners met regularly to plan curriculum and the delivery of the program. There was intentional overlap between groups. Much of the work of the teams was accomplished via teleconference and e-mail communication because of scheduling demands and geographic separation. A description of the EBP portion of the overall curriculum is delineated in **Box 1**.

The program was inspired by the existence of gaps in linkages between clinical information systems, best EBP interventions, and nursing-sensitive patient quality outcomes. The curriculum was designed to bridge the knowledge gaps between these areas and to provide participants with the leadership skills vital for transforming their learning into sustainable practice innovations. Because of the number of metrics included in the NQF nursing-sensitive measure set, it was decided that only one NQF measure would be used as an exemplar for each NQF scholar cohort to unify effort and learning using one specific clinical issue. The objective was to teach specific skills that then could be generalized when approaching other nursing-sensitive measures.

DESCRIPTION OF THE INTENDED PARTICIPANTS

Candidates were identified by the chief nurse executive in each of the participating organizations and had nurse manager support for participation. Nurses were recruited based on their interest and commitment to the yearlong program as well as on their leadership potential. Individuals who currently were in leadership positions and desired the expanded knowledge in the curricular content as well as nurses who showed promise in becoming enduring change agents and who had informal and/or formal leadership influence were prime applicants.

In year one (2007–2008), 51 nurses from across all sites participated with a focus on hospital-based nursing. In year two (2008–2009), an additional 40 nurses from across all sites were enrolled, and the focus was on clinic-, homecare-, and long-term care–based nursing. The number of nurses recruited for the project depended on availability and workload at their respective sites.

PROGRAM IMPLEMENTATION

The program began in the winter with an orientation meeting at the most central and largest site within the system. In a face-to-face session participants were introduced to the components of the NQF Scholars Program and became aware of resources,

---

Box 1
EBP content outline

1. Discuss the history of EBP

2. Discuss goals and processes of EBP as compared with the conduct of nursing research and nursing quality initiatives

3. Outline the importance of EBP to professional nursing practice in terms of the American Nurses Association Social Policy Statement

4. Describe the use of evidence in achieving positive NQF outcomes

5. Formulate a clinical/educational or administrative question using a structured format

6. Identify accurate search strategies and applicable databases for addressing evidence-based nursing practice questions

7. Select research articles applicable to the clinical question from the library search.

8. Practice skills for evaluating and critiquing individual research articles and groups of articles.

9. Practice skills of literature synthesis verbally and in writing, assessing levels and quality of evidence.

10. Evaluate and compare published guidelines.

11. Select the appropriate outcome measure (evaluation of published scales).

12. Critique systematic reviews.

13. Apply the process of critically appraising the literature into a "clinical bottom line."

14. Describe conceptual and implementation models that guide evidence-based nursing practice.

15. Describe how theories of change and diffusion of innovation can be used to support EBP.

16. Describe implementation strategies.

17. Identify specific organizational, provider, and patient barriers and facilitators to implementing EBP processes and policies.

18. Describe feasible evaluation frameworks for selected EBP initiatives.

19. Identify ways that leadership strategies can be combined with EBP methods to ensure translation of evidence in to practice in an effective and sustainable fashion.

20. Describe how to evaluate a practice change and know that it is sustainable.

---

such as online learning tools and library services. NQF scholars were provided an overview that included an orientation to clinical informatics, the basics of NQF quality metrics, and fundamental elements of EBP. The second day, participants attended a Nursing Research Conference that focused on EBP.

The initial 10-week content session was an online graduate course on clinical informatics offered through the Oregon Health and Science University in partnership with the American Medical Informatics Association (AMIA), an AMIA 10 × 10 program that emphasizes EBP.[11] The informatics coursework was concluded when the NQF scholars came back to the central site for a 2-day face-to-face meeting. During this meeting, the faculty for the EBP course introduced the curriculum outline and provided the first module of content. Delivery method of the 12-module EBP course primarily was online asynchronously, with some synchronous meetings available as well. All sessions were recorded to allow later playback.

Because the curriculum was designed with the NQF metrics in mind, one metric of interest was chosen for all of the scholars to work on for the remainder of the course: the incidence and point prevalence of pressure ulcers for cohort one and the prevalence of falls and of falls with injury for cohort two. The scholars also received a summer assignment designed to help them learn more about local resources and personnel involved with informatics, EBP, and quality initiatives (see Appendix). The intention behind this assignment was to lighten the workload for the scholars at this point in the curriculum and to achieve a connection with quality improvements already occurring in their respective sites.

The next face-to-face meeting occurred in the fall when the scholars had completed several EBP modules. A module was delivered during a 2-day meeting, and work sessions were offered for online scholarly inquiry. Groups of scholars formed to work on various projects related to pressure ulcers. Content was delivered during this 2-day meeting on quality methodologies, human factors, leadership, and project development.

After the EBP modules were completed, the scholar groups continued to meet locally to incorporate content from the EBP course along with informatics and quality measures into their pressure ulcer projects. In the mid-winter a virtual meeting was arranged between the scholars and some of the faculty so that the scholars could report on the progress of the pressure ulcer-related EBP projects and quality initiatives and the faculty could provide leadership and mentorship content formally. A secondary outcome of these presentations was the excitement of learning about different products sites were using for pressure ulcers and the possibility of purchasing these products for the other sites as well as the recognition of the work that had been accomplished thus far.

In the spring, the first cohort of scholars met for their final planned face-to-face meeting to celebrate their accomplishments, to initiate mentoring work with the second cohort of NQF scholars who were in the initial phase of their curriculum, and to develop plans for sustaining their knowledge and skills. This meeting intentionally coincided with a large, system-wide quality conference that held many opportunities for participant networking and communicating about the NQF Scholars Program with other disciplines. Virtual seminars are planned quarterly to sustain the ongoing work of the first cohort of NQF scholars.

CASE EXAMPLES: NQF SCHOLAR EVIDENCE-BASED PRACTICE PROJECT TEAMS

As described earlier in this article, the NQF scholars formed local work groups that focused on specific, local clinical issues relevant to the assessment, prevention, or treatment of pressure ulcers. The teams formulated a question using the population of interest/intervention of interest/comparative intervention/outcome (PICO) format, searched and synthesized the pertinent literature, and designed a plan to translate the evidence into nursing practice. The results of the literature synthesis were used in various ways, including being posted on the shared drive for use by all NQF scholar groups. Also, the work of the groups has been used to inform and guide the enterprise-wide pressure ulcer initiative. Local efforts have varied and continue to emerge. Specific examples of clinical questions that were identified by the NQF scholar groups are

- How does nursing knowledge affect early recognition of pressure ulcers?
- Will providing a standardized education program for patients and families decrease the incidence of preventable pressure ulcers?
- In immobile, bedridden patients, does the use of Granulex help prevent skin breakdown?

- Does a Web-based teaching module with hyperlinked video recordings increase interrater and intrarater reliability among staff nurses and wound, osteotomy, and continence nurses for differentiating pressure ulcers from moisture-associated skin lesions?
- Is there an instrument (incorporating oxygenation perfusion and/or fluid balance) that is more accurate than the Braden Scale for Predicting Pressure Sore Risk in assessing risk for developing pressure ulcers in critically ill patients?
- In hospitalized patients at risk for developing pressure ulcers, do "just in time" electronic reminders decrease the incidence of pressure ulcers as compared with current practice?
- In adult hospitalized patients, is the Braden Scale for Predicting Pressure Sore Risk the most effective scoring instrument for assessing the risk of developing pressure ulcers?

The group projects often resulted in the scholars accessing all the three major curricular areas of informatics, EBP, and nursing-sensitive measures. In the words of one NQF scholar,

Our local project focused around the evidence on pressure ulcer risk assessment scales. In examining how we were using informatics to assist with our project, we discovered that reports were being generated weekly related to pressure ulcers. As we progressed through the project, the group sought out other ideas in how to use an electronic health record. In the future, we would like to incorporate decision support for the nursing staff when documenting on pressure ulcers – such as recommended interventions that are based on the best evidence.

LEADERSHIP/MENTORSHIP

The systematic translation of best evidence into clinical practice was a primary overarching goal of the NQF Scholars Program, particularly the EBP component. Content knowledge and EBP skills are critical in attaining this goal, but they are not sufficient to initiate and sustain meaningful change; leadership skills are required to gain momentum to initiate, implement, evaluate, and sustain practice innovations. Likewise, clinical informatics and quality improvement initiatives are successful both because individuals have the cognitive skills in place and because leaders have exerted effective influence to make enduring changes in practice. Nurses at all levels of the system are considered leaders. Therefore, the development of leadership skills was included in the program content. Leadership was introduced in the first face-to-face meeting and was included in the EBP modules. During the final session, cohorts one and two had the opportunity to participate in a "speed mentoring" activity designed to initiate mentoring relationships between the cohorts. In this exercise cohort two participants had a short, timed (3 minutes) chance to interact with cohort one participants to investigate possible opportunities for shared learning or mentoring. The activity was completed in a lighthearted but focused manner.

CHALLENGES

Transitioning from a focus on the individual organization to a system-wide scope brought new challenges and opportunities. Providing education and support in a health care system–wide manner expanded the capacity for organizational learning and also presented new complexities that were distinct from previous hospital- and clinic-based approaches. These challenges, opportunities, and complexities, along with suggestions for future directions are discussed here.

First, the program participants were geographically dispersed across the Southeast, Southwest, and Midwest areas of the continental United States. Participants were in different time zones, different organizational structures and cultures, and various communication systems. Participants came from varied clinical settings and roles with widely differing responsibilities and reporting structures. To address this challenge, a great deal of flexibility was built into the educational delivery system. Web-based formats were used whenever possible, and distinct individual modules that could be accessed in a variety of settings were provided. Because the participants worked in the same system but in different locations, there was the benefit of a common infrastructure and support network for computer access and Web-based technologies. A second strategy for meeting this challenge was providing periodic face-to-face meetings at the most central location so that participants would have the opportunity to get to know each other, develop relationships, and network. Many of the instructional modules were provided in asynchronous formats, but several synchronous sessions also were posted in the spirit of "office hours" so that participants could ask questions of the instructor and project planners in a real-time format.

Another challenge in program delivery was that the participants had various levels of clinical expertise and different educational backgrounds, many of which did not include EBP or research coursework. Some participants came from organizations with strong nursing research and EBP infrastructures and processes in place; other nurses had access to more limited resources. To address the issue of varied preparation, the course was designed at the postgraduate level, but resources for more basic content areas were available. Textbooks on EBP and nursing research were provided for each participant as reference resources. In addition, project planners and faculty were available by e-mail and telephone for questions and assistance. Web-based resources also were made available, and a tutorial regarding electronically available library resources was included in one of the face-to-face sessions. In many cases, nurses who were more expert in EBP or in critiquing and using research in practice paired with more novice participants to help them understand the concepts. The major project was accomplished in a group setting to facilitate informal mentoring and to maximize the expertise of all members.

Participants not only came from diverse geographic settings and educational backgrounds; they also represented varied clinical positions and professional roles. This variety presented a challenge in crafting the curriculum and assignments in a way that would be pertinent to every participant, but the situation also had advantages, because participants could view issues from a variety of perspectives. Part of the EBP course was a group project focused on the development of a PICO question, appropriate search and critique of the literature, design of a synthesis table, and formulation of an implementation plan. The project groups met the challenges of diversity by optimizing the positives: coordinating schedules, using asynchronous communication (usually e-mail), and using each other's unique strengths. Group members had to keep themselves and each other accountable for group assignments.

A major challenge for the faculty and participants was the ability to tie the three domains of EBP, clinical informatics, and nursing-sensitive quality measures together in a meaningful way, regardless of clinical role of the participant. Within the curriculum, threads of statistical methods, leadership skills, and Web-based tools also were woven across the three major content domains. It was important that the curricular domains were standardized in their delivery but flexible enough to accommodate diffusion of innovation within several different organizational cultures represented by the nurses from different sites. Much of the program content synthesis remained to be evaluated formally at the end of the 1-year program, but participants anecdotally reported that they were starting to see ways that they could integrate EBP, clinical informatics, and nursing quality metrics into their everyday work processes. For example, one NQF scholar group began formal meetings with their local hospital-based wound ostomy nursing team to disseminate the synthesized literature about the pressure ulcer severity rating system currently in use. Additionally, participants noted that they were more aware of the presence of these content areas in their practice, although they might not have been attuned to them before participating in the program.

Perhaps one of the most challenging aspects of the program was the short timeline for implementing the curriculum. Internal funding was received for the 2-year project, and work began immediately to put together the curriculum and instructional delivery systems. The compressed timeframe led the faculty and planning team to be focused and innovative in their approaches and to use time wisely. The faculty and steering group wanted the content for all three areas to be rigorous and externally valid, so a variety of academic programs and providers was explored. For the EBP portion of the curriculum, it was important to provide content that was theoretically grounded, that had scholarly merit and clear clinical relevance, and that highlighted the role of the direct-care nurse in leading EBP initiatives with institutional support. Fortunately, the EBP course and the clinical informatics course were available from external entities; the organization contracted with these individuals and organizations to provide the content, while the faculty and planners managed the delivery and coordination of the curriculum. Formative curriculum and evaluation strategies are in place to modify the curriculum for subsequent cohorts. Adaptations will include integrating the content more completely across modules, sustaining collaborative work groups that emphasize EBP, and more completely introducing and reinforcing leadership content within the program.

In the future, efforts for leadership and mentorship education will be more explicit, systematic, and intentional. Expectations that scholars will pursue leadership, mentorship, and a sustained scholarship role as a result of the program will be expressed and reinforced from the beginning and will be integrated into follow-up online working groups. Even though leadership potential was among the criteria for participation in the program, some participants came into the program with strong leadership skills, and others were relative novices. In retrospect, leadership training is an aspect of the program that could be strengthened in the future. There is great untapped potential in arranging the sharing of leadership skills among scholars at different levels of experience and expertise across the system. Leadership skills are likely to play a key role in program sustainability.

FACILITATING FACTORS

Many factors worked together to make this initiative successful. The program had organizational support from the highest levels of administration that translated into endorsement, time allocation, and financial resources. At every level a high value was placed on developing nursing workforce knowledge and competencies for future generations of the nursing profession. The benefits were articulated in potential impact on outcomes of patient care (safety, effectiveness, and quality) and in workforce optimization (nursing satisfaction, retention, and professional development).

Fiscal resources were critical in providing time for the nurses to participate, including travel expenses to attend all-site meetings, curricular fees for the content provided, textbooks, and online educational support. Personnel resources for a project planning team consisted of three individuals who coordinated participant communication and enrollment, provided meeting schedules and agendas, managed the instructional design and technology resources, and provided administrative oversight of the continuing education aspects of the program. Continuing education units were awarded to participants, and one of the program planners served as coordinator of this process. Program faculty scheduled time to meet, plan, and evaluate the curriculum as it was developed.

High levels of motivation and expertise of participants and faculty served as catalysts for program implementation. The organization had access to information technology expertise and resources that facilitated the actual delivery of the education and helped bridge the geographic distance among participants. Fortunately, recognized experts in the content areas were available both within the system and from highly respected external entities. Faculty members had broad professional networks on which to draw when planning how the content areas should be provided.

LESSONS LEARNED

Many valuable lessons emerged.

- The project planning team was vital in meeting the timeframes of the program and for coordinating workflows.
- Face-to-face meetings with participants, planning team, and faculty were important for building connections, networking, developing leadership skills, and conveying the larger context of the work.
- Choosing a clinically relevant issue (eg, pressure ulcers) as the focus for the EBP projects served to unify the work of the clinically diverse nurse participants.
- Work groups helped participants divide the effort and understand how to make it most meaningful clinically.
- The diverse roles of participants were turned into a benefit: sharing complementary expertise.
- Work groups sometimes met virtually because of scheduling challenges. This practice was not always ideal, but technology support helped greatly.
- The instruction was available online through a shared portal server (Sharepoint) and a meeting/educational delivery application (Interwise), so it was possible for geographically dispersed participants to interact effectively.
- The compressed timeframe for the curriculum kept the momentum going, but participants sometimes needed more time to synthesize their learning and translate it in clinically meaningful ways.
- Participants expressed the need for consistently communicated expectations regarding the time and resources needed to complete assignments.
- There was a need for stronger and more formal preparation for leadership/ change agent portion of the curriculum. Even with the best EBP content, strong leadership skills are essential to bring about practice transformation based on best evidence.
- Participants valued faculty presence and availability.
- The outcomes and future roles sometimes were vague. There was not always a definite answer to the question, "How will I use this in my job right now?"
- There was a need to manage, incorporate, and treat the modules as an integrated curriculum; the three content areas are not "plug and play."
- Setting participant expectations was very important; an identified need was to build in a spirit of comfort with ambiguity and preparation for an unknown and largely unpredictable future, because nursing roles are evolving constantly.

SUMMARY AND CONCLUSIONS

This article has described the implementation of a system-wide curriculum for nurses incorporating the content domains of informatics, EBP, and quality methodologies focused on a nursing-sensitive performance measure set. Transitioning the focus from individual organization to a system-wide approach meant that the implementation required innovative strategies to optimize outcomes despite disparate geographic locations, nursing education, and professional expertise of the participants. The diversity of the participants greatly enriched the outcomes of the program, both in the projects that were designed and in the collegial relationships that were formed. The system-wide approach was facilitated by the resources of time, technology, personnel expertise, rigorous course content, and leadership support across the system. Future challenges include making the program sustainable for the long term, developing leadership content and teaching modalities that meet varying levels of learner need, completing formal evaluations of the curriculum and outcomes, and discerning which components of the program are best suited for different nurse constituents.

APPENDIX. DEPARTMENT OF NURSING NQF SCHOLARS PROGRAM SUMMER ASSIGNMENT
Purposes

There are three purposes for this summer assignment: (1) to begin to establish dialogues and relationships within each site related to data, evidence-based practice, and the NQF nurse-sensitive measure set; (2) to begin to create a bridge between the didactic content from the informatics module to the data activities that enable collection of NQF nurse-sensitive measures, and (3) to lay a foundation for the evidence-based practice content that will start in the late summer.

Assignment

First, meet with the Chief Nursing Officer at your site and identify a plan for meeting with key stakeholders (eg, quality department, practice committees, and others) to identify the key efforts at your site related to data sources for the NQF nurse-sensitive measures, the underlying practices that are associated with the NQF nurse-sensitive measures, and any technologies that are used at your site that contain information related to NQF nurse-sensitive measures or the practices you might associate with an NQF nurse-sensitive measure.

Example

One of the NQF nurse-sensitive measures is concerned with the point prevalence of pressure ulcers. It would be helpful if you could determine how data about pressure ulcers are collected at your site. Who combines that data across units? What types of order sets or practice guidelines did you previously identify related to pressure ulcers at your site? Try to connect with the individual or group working on that order set. Ask whether the data are being converted to an electronic format and if information will be included in the electronic medical record. Find out who is submitting information about pressure ulcers to various reporting groups (including NQF nursing measures). Are there individuals and/or committees working on best practices concerning pressure ulcers?

The questions in **Table 2** are intended as sample questions to help you get the dialogue started.

Table 2		
Examples of Contacts	**Sample Discussion Topics/Questions You Might Ask the Contact Person**	**Notes**
Chief nursing officer	What are we doing with the NQF nurse-sensitive measures we are currently collecting? My expectations/ideals about the NQF scholars program are [fill in the blank!]. What are your expectations of my involvement in this program? Do you see overlap between the NQF nurse-sensitive measures and other quality and evidence-based projects? Do you see opportunities for information technologies to enhance the capture of data related to NQF measures? What opportunities do you see for information technologies to enhance specific areas of our practice? Who would you suggest I talk with this summer so that I can get a more complete picture of the connection between quality measures, the NQF nurse-sensitive measures (specifically, evidence-based and best practices), and the use of information technology to support?	
Staff that work with quality initiatives (within nursing and for your institution)	In what ways do the NQF nurse-sensitive measures overlap with other measures currently being collected in the organization? How are the data for NQF measures being collected? Who is collecting the data? What electronic systems are used throughout the collection, analysis, and reporting NQF nurse-sensitive and related measures? Is a quality model used in our quality department?	
Information technology staff	How do you identify what vocabulary or terminology to use when developing or modifying applications?	
Practice analysts	Is much modification of applications done here? If so, how do you get a sense of the business need for making those modifications?	
Informatics staff	How do you develop an understanding of the process flows that need to be supported in specific applications? Is there a template or standard set of information that would be useful for you to have before engaging in conversations with clinicians about software modifications? How are priorities set for information technology at our site?	
Other persons or roles that may assist in projects (eg, nursing and medicine practice colleagues)	Do we have project managers? How do you organize to "get the work done" on a specific project? How would you recommend I go about identifying key stakeholders for any practice project?	

REFERENCES

1. National Quality Forum (NQF). National voluntary consensus standards for nursing-sensitive care: an initial performance measure set. Washington, DC: NQF;2004. Available at: http://www.qualityforum.org/pdf/nursing-quality/txNCFINALpublic.pdf. Accessed May 20, 2008.
2. Tucker S, Derscheid D, Odegarden S, et al. Evidence based training for enhancing psychiatric nurses' child behavior management skills. J Nurses Staff Dev 2008; 24(2):75–85.
3. Neumann J, Brady-Schluttner K, Street W. Developing nursing scholars: implementation of a multi-faceted, integrated staff development project. Presented at the Second Annual National Database Of Nursing Quality Indicators Conference. Orlando, January 30–February 1, 2008.
4. Neumann J, Brady-Schluttner, Timm J. Nursing professionalism: accountablity and image. National Quality Forum Scholars Program poster presentation, Mayo Clinic Rochester. Rochester, April 8, 2008.
5. Neumann J, Brady-Schluttner K. NQF scholars engaging in excellence in nursing practice. A journey. Defining Excellence Magnet ANCC National Magnet Conference. October 15–17, 2008.
6. Pipe T, Cisar N, Caruso E, et al. Leadership strategies: inspiring evidence-based practice at the organizational and unit levels. J Nurs Care Qual 2008;23(3): 266–72.
7. Pipe T. Optimizing nursing care by integrating theory-driven evidence-based practice. Journal of Nursing Care Quality 2007;22(3):234–8.
8. Pipe T, Wellik K, Buchda V, et al. Implementing evidence-based nursing practice. Med Surg Nursing 2005;14(3):179–84.
9. Schultz A. Clinical scholars at the bedside: an EBP mentorship model for today. Online Journal of Excellence in Nursing Knowledge. Available at: http://www.nursingknowledge.org. Accessed May 28, 2008.
10. Institute of Medicine, Keeping patients safe: transforming the work environment of nurses, committee on the work environment for nurses and patient safety, Page A (ed.). Institute of Medicine of the National Academies, 2004. The National Academies Press, Washington, DC Available at: www.nap.edu. Accessed May 20, 2008.
11. American Medical Association of Informatics web site. Available at: http://www.amia.org/10x10. Accessed, May 20, 2008.

Promotion of Safe Outcomes: Incorporating Evidence into Policies and Procedures

Lisa English Long, MSN, RN, CNS*, Karen Burkett, MS, RN, CNP,
Susan McGee, MSN, RN, CNP

KEYWORDS

• Evidence • Policies • Procedures • Outcomes • Safety

Policies and procedures (P&Ps) provide guidance in the care nurses provide to patients and families. The goal of achieving safe practice can be obtained through the use of P&Ps. To further enhance the effect of P&Ps on patient care, incorporation of evidence provides documentation of safe and best practice. The addition of evidence to P&Ps requires the development of a process to ensure consistency, rigor, and safe nursing practice.

This article describes the process of incorporating evidence into P&Ps, resulting in the establishment of evidence as a basis for safe practice. The process described includes use of the Rosswurm and Larrabee[1] model for change to evidence-based practice. The model guided the work of evidence-based practice mentors in developing a template, system, and educational plan for dissemination of evidence-based P&Ps into patient care.

ASSESS

Point-of-care nurses focus on the use of current best evidence to guide their practice. Caring for patients also involves the use of P&Ps, which provide the direction to implement procedures, patient education, and evaluation of interventions in an approach that focuses on safety. For P&Ps to be based on best practice, evidence must be integrated. The addition of evidence to P&Ps requires the development of a process to ensure consistency, rigor, and safe nursing practice.

Evidence-Based Practice, Center for Professional Excellence-Research and Evidence-Based Practice, Cincinnati Children's Hospital Medical Center, 3333 Burnett Avenue, ML 11016, Cincinnati, OH 45229, USA
* Corresponding author.
E-mail address: lisa.long@cchmc.org (L.E. Long).

Nurs Clin N Am 44 (2009) 57–70
doi:10.1016/j.cnur.2008.10.013
0029-6465/08/$ – see front matter © 2009 Elsevier Inc. All rights reserved.

To ensure integration of evidence in the P&Ps of a large midwestern pediatric academic medical center, evidence-based practice mentors were charged with reviewing, updating, and incorporating evidence into 32 P&Ps over a 6-month time frame. Within the medical center, evidence-based practice mentors are advanced practice nurses with additional education in evidence-based practice. The focus of the mentors is to collaborate with nursing staff in addressing clinical issues. The role of the mentors involves education, facilitation, implementation, and evaluation of evidence in practice. The mentors within this organization have approached evidence work from a unit-based and systems perspective.

To begin the assessment phase, internal and external data about current practices were gathered to determine organizational readiness for change to an evidence-based P&P process. The institution did not at this point have a clear definition of evidence-based policies or procedures. Within the institution, definitions of policy, procedure, and standard were inconsistent from policy manual to policy manual and from division to division.

Internal to the organization, within the nursing division, multiple online policy manuals were used by staff. These manuals were selected from nursing divisional policy manuals and critical care unit manuals. The nursing P&P manual for the division included over 100 P&Ps. Policy manuals within the many critical care units often included a greater number of P&Ps than in the divisional manual. In each of the P&Ps, references were noted; however, the references were not leveled and graded. To provide a logical starting point, senior nursing leadership determined early that the focus of the work would be to evidence base the divisional nursing P&P manual.

Internal data suggested an auspicious approach to implementing a change. First, there was recognition from the senior leadership team that policies based on evidence would sustain best practices, promote improved patient outcomes, and were a necessary requirement for Magnet recognition. Second, with support from senior leadership, the divisional Nurse Practice Council (NPC) adopted a goal to evidence base P&Ps but struggled with how to operationalize that goal. Third, the evidence-based practice mentor team, who were asked to lead this process, recognized that "evidence-based policies are outcomes that can be derived from the EBP process."[2]

External data included reports from the Institute of Medicine that supported the proposed change. At a national level, the Institute of Medicine reports discussed the importance of safety in health care and the use of evidence in decision making within the practice arena.[3] In discussions with health care organizations about the use of evidence within P&Ps, the evidence-based practice mentor team noted that inconsistencies existed, especially in the referencing and leveling and grading of the evidence. Most institutions used either textbooks or published procedure manuals for a reference to provide some evidence for procedural policies. Overall, those references were not leveled and graded.

LINK

Evidence-based practice mentors addressed the rationale for the aspiration to develop P&Ps based on evidence. The vision and mission of the organization's focus on safety and best practice and the institution's current Magnet journey supported the need for evidence to be integrated into P&Ps.

Linking the problem of a lack of evaluated evidence embedded in policy to measurable outcomes was a critical element in this process. Outcomes are often defined within the all-encompassing concepts of patient, nurse, cost, and organizational effects. Identifying an outcome that was specific and measurable was needed to drive the process of incorporating evidence into nursing practice. The recent attention at this institution to the National Patient Safety Initiatives[4] guided the evidence-based practice mentor team to patient safety. Patient safety outcomes became the focal point around which all clinical questions were centered.

To reach the desired outcomes, the five steps of evidence-based practice were used as a guide to the evidence process.[2] These steps include the following:

1. Asking the burning clinical questions
2. Collecting the most relevant and best evidence
3. Critically appraising the evidence
4. Integrating all evidence with one's clinical expertise, patient preferences, and values in making a practice decision or change
5. Evaluating the practice decision or change

Use of these steps guided formulation of the clinical question, the search for evidence, and evaluation of the evidence to make a recommendation relevant to each policy or procedure reviewed. These steps also informed the evaluation of the proposed process of embedding evidence into P&Ps.

SYNTHESIS

The five steps of evidence-based practice were a model for the evidence work guided and facilitated by the evidence-based practice mentors. The mentors engaged in the process of designing a change so that P&Ps were based on evidence. The standardized language of PICO (population, intervention, comparison, outcome) was used to formulate the clinical question "Among nurses, does the use of evidence versus traditional care improve patient safety outcomes?"

Systematic search strategies were employed including multiple databases and key words pertinent to the PICO question. Databases searched included CINAHL, PubMed, Medline, and the National Guidelines Clearinghouse. Search terms were *nurses*, *patients*, *safety*, and *improved outcomes*.

Findings from the literature search and subsequent evidence review demonstrated positive outcomes such as improved staff satisfaction,[5] patient care,[6] and cost outcomes[7] when using evidence in clinical practice; however, no research studies related to the general concept of patient safety and the use of evidence were found. Although it may be implied that improved safety can result from using evidence in practice, it has not been studied. The National Patient Safety Initiatives[4] suggest that patient safety improves with the use of evidence in practice. In addition, third party payers request evidence to support reimbursement provided to health care organizations for patient care. The answer to the clinical question was "When nurses use evidence versus traditional care in clinical practice, many nurse satisfaction, cost, and patient care outcomes are improved." No research findings supported the use of evidence to improve patient safety. Although research is needed in the area of safety, the research evidence related to satisfaction, cost, and patient care outcomes plus the clinical expertise related to safety support the concept of embedding evidence into P&Ps.

DESIGN

The proposed change would lead to the integration of evidence into 32 divisional nursing P&Ps. To accomplish the change to evidence-based P&Ps, a well-defined process was needed to maintain consistency within the work led by the evidence-based practice mentors. To initiate this process, the evidence-based practice mentor team defined "evidence-based P&Ps" as P&Ps supported by leveled and graded references, with a clinical question focusing on the safety of each policy or procedure. The revised or new P&Ps included a recommendation based on a safety-related evidence search, appraisal, and synthesis.

To begin the process, identification of an evidence-based procedure book that could serve as the main reference for the nursing division's P&P manual was undertaken by the evidence-based practice mentors. The goal was to identify a procedure manual with integrated evidence. Mentors identified stakeholders to serve on the team to review and recommend a manual, including point-of-care staff accountable for the P&Ps. A nine-member point-of-care review team was composed of point-of-care nurses, a medical librarian, and evidence-based practice mentors. This team rated online pediatric evidence-based procedure manuals. A textbook evaluation instrument[8] had been adapted for use in evaluating pediatric content, online format, and evidence-based qualities of nursing procedure manuals. Through the use of this instrument, one manual was selected from three that were reviewed.

The selection of a procedure manual with integrated evidence provided guidance in integrating evidence within P&Ps. It was imperative that references listed within the chosen manual had been reviewed in a rigorous process that included the leveling of each study and grading of the body of evidence. When this did not appear in the manual, the institutional definition of evidence-based P&P provided guidance and clarification.

The next action needed to attain the outcome of evidence-based P&Ps was the development of a template to provide a consistent format. To address this need, a leadership group was formed consisting of senior nursing leaders, legal services, NPC leaders, policy and procedure committee members, and the evidence-based practice mentor team. The template format was similar to the previously used process for organizing P&Ps. The key difference was the availability of current, synthesized evidence related to pertinent safety issues of each policy or procedure. A supplementary document template was developed to maintain a record of the review date and process. This template included the names of the review team members, the reference list with levels, the grade of the body of evidence, the recommendation for practice based on the evidence review, and a key to the appraisal system used (**Box 1**).

In addition to the policy name, number, and date of origin and review, the template includes five main headings: policy, purpose, guideline for procedure, references, and implementation. The template includes cues to the definitions of the headings and the information that should be included under each one. The "policy" heading cue indicates that this section answers the question "What is this policy (procedure)?" This section defines who is licensed to enact the policy or to perform the procedure.

Box 1
Summary of nursing policy, procedure, and standards review process

Policy #/Name:

Review Team:

PICO Question:

References (with Level & Grade):

    (Level __ Evidence)

    [Strength of the Body of Evidence as of (most recent review date): Grade]

Courtesy of EBP Mentor Team, Cincinnati Children's Hospital Medical Center, Cincinnati, OH; with permission. Copyright, © 2007, EBP Mentor Team.

The "purpose" heading cue is the question "Why does this policy exist?" The team considers if there is a regulatory, safety, or process requirement for the topic under consideration. If not, a recommendation might be made to the pertinent committee to delete the policy or procedure. If the group determines there is a need, this section of the template includes the aim of the P&P or the desired outcome.

The "guideline for the procedure" provides the steps that are required to perform an activity, answering the question "How do I follow this policy?" If there is a corresponding procedure in the online procedure manual, a link to that procedure is created. Any recommended variation to the online procedure is identified by a symbol inserted into the relevant document. If there is no corresponding online procedure, the steps to perform the procedure are listed within the policy or procedure template.

The fourth heading in the template is the "reference" list. Identification of the quality level of the individual article is noted at the end of each citation, answering the question "Is the study valid, reliable, and applicable to the population of interest?" At the end of the reference list, the review team provides a grade for the body of the evidence and answers the question "What are the quality, quantity, and consistency of the evidence that speaks to the PICO question?" Tables of the quality level and grading systems are included within the template.

The final template heading of "implementation" addresses how the policy or procedure will be implemented. The intention of this heading is to answer the question "Who is responsible for this policy?" For example, nursing procedures are typically maintained by the NPC. If a policy affects more than one discipline, the responsible group would be the Interdisciplinary Practice Committee. Minimally, P&Ps are reviewed every 3 years. If a need to make a change based on new research evidence occurs, a practitioner brings this to the attention of the responsible group for earlier review. This process can be initiated by any staff member, beginning the task of developing evidence-based P&Ps.

In addition, the template includes reference lists with each reference leveled and graded. When using the accepted manual or online resources, it was noted that many resources did not engage in the rigorous process of leveling each study and grading a body of evidence. This discovery led to the definition of an evidence-based policy or procedure that raised the standard for evidence evaluation. The development of a template supported the definition of an evidence-based P&P as a policy or procedure that was focused on patient safety. In addition, the goal for the evidence to be leveled and graded was evident within the template. This definition made explicit three key components: (1) the focus of the evidence search and evaluation would be patient safety outcomes; (2) the evidence would be leveled and graded for quality, quantity, and consistency of the findings; and (3) the strength of the evidence would provide a recommendation to support or refute the need for a change in practice.

Successful template development led to a systematic selection of 32 P&Ps for revision or development by point-of-care review teams. P&Ps were grouped by clinical area or condition (eg, all policies on documentation or all procedures related to vascular access) and divided among the evidence-based practice mentors. The mentors had the primary responsibility for overseeing completion of the evidence work on each of the 32 policies. Grouping of related policies or procedures allowed the evidence-based practice mentors to identify evidence that overlapped and consider consolidation of P&Ps if appropriate. For example, if there was strong evidence of the effectiveness of chlorhexidine gluconate to reduce infections for central venous catheters and peripheral intravenous catheters, the evidence could be embedded in each procedure.

This phase of the practice change outlined a "sequence of activities in a descriptive format."[1] The sequenced actions were set in motion once the point-of-care review teams were formed. The teams would begin a review of the current policy or procedure and weigh it against the procedure from the manual with integrated evidence. If there were slight changes needed to the policy, it could be customized for current practice and the evidence embedded with references that were leveled and graded. For online procedures that required small changes, a link to the online procedure reference was provided; however, if too many amendments were required to the online procedure manual, it was abandoned, and the P&P template was used independently to construct a new policy or procedure. In an effort to keep the policy or procedure concise, the supplementary document was used to summarize the policy or procedure review process.

When the mentors had lists of P&Ps for review, each identified the appropriate stakeholders for every topic and formed P&P review teams. These teams were comprised of clinicians familiar with the policy or procedure based on their use within the clinical setting. Nursing staff accountable for the practice guided by that procedure or policy were the obvious choice for review team members. Others potential review team members were advanced practice nurses, clinical managers, education coordinators, or outcome managers. The purpose of the additional clinical staff was the expertise they offered in relation to the P&P under review. The evidence-based practice mentors as part of the team located and evaluated the evidence. The team reviewed the revised P&P for accuracy, clarity, and applicability to practice.

In support of the shared governance structure within the organization, upon completion of the P&P, one of the evidence-based practice mentors would forward the P&P in the new template along with the supplementary document to the divisional NPC. The NPC would review the document and approve it for placement within the P&P manual.

Table 1	
Sample of policies and procedures with clinical questions	
Policy or Procedure Name	**PICO Question Related to Patient Safety**
Policy	
Bed placement	Among hospitalized children, does restriction of co-bedding versus co-bedding of adults and children reduce the risk of suffocation or injury?
Patient classification system	Among hospital nurses, does use of a patient classification system tool increase safety and effectiveness in staffing standards?
Student nurses	In providing care to pediatric patients, does allowing nursing students to administer medications lead to an increase in medication errors versus medication errors among experienced nurses?
Procedure	
Central venous catheters	Among hospitalized children, does use of chlorhexidine gluconate scrub versus Betadine and alcohol scrub decrease the incidence of catheter-related infections?
Intramuscular injections	Among infants requiring an intramuscular injection, does use of a long needle versus short needle reduce localized reactions?
Healing touch	For hospitalized children, does the use of healing touch by certified healing touch practitioners have any adverse effects compared with hospitalized children who are not treated with healing touch?

Table 2 Levels of evidence	
Level	**Description**
I	Systematic review or meta-analysis of RCTs or evidence-based practice guidelines based on RCTs
II	At least one well-designed RCT
III	Well-designed controlled trials without randomization (quasi-experimental)
IV	Well-designed case-control and cohort studies
V	Systematic reviews of descriptive and qualitative studies
VI	One descriptive or qualitative study
VII	Expert opinion or reports of expert committees

Abbreviation: RCT, randomized controlled trial.
Adapted from Melnyk BM, Fineout-Overholt E. Evidence-based practice in nursing & healthcare: a guide to best practice. Philadelphia: Lippincott; 2005; with permission.

To introduce the new process of embedding evidence into P&Ps to the nursing staff, an educational plan was developed by the mentors in collaboration with leadership of the NPC. The education was provided to members of NPC and to the nurse educators group, unit-based educators responsible for communicating and educating staff about practice changes on each unit.

IMPLEMENTATION

Implementation of the new process began with the evidence-based practice mentors identifying the 32 P&Ps to be reviewed. The online procedure manual had been selected by the nine-member point-of-care review team.

For the manual to reflect the practice in a consistent manner, the template developed by the leadership group was used with each P&P under review. This template was the blueprint for the content and format of evidence-based P&Ps. Using the template, evidence-based policies or procedures were developed that ranged from policies on bed placement and patient classification systems to procedures on central venous catheters and healing touch.

With the systems and process developed, synthesizing the evidence for the P&Ps commenced. This step meant finding answers to the clinical questions formulated from key patient safety concerns for each policy or procedure (**Table 1**). "The purpose

Box 2 Grading the strength of the body of evidence
A. Level I evidence
B. Consistent findings from levels II, III, IV, or V
C. Inconsistent findings from levels II, III, IV, or V
D. Little or no evidence or level VI only
E. Level VII

Data from Schiffer CA, Anderson K, Bennett C, et al. ASCO special article. Platelet transfusion for patients with cancer: clinical practice guidelines of the American Society of Clinical Oncology. J Clin Oncol 2001;19(5):1519–38.

Table 3
Integrated table (evidence summary) for PICO question "Among pediatric hospitalized patients requiring a central venous catheter, does use of chlorhexidine gluconate scrub versus Betadine and alcohol scrub decrease the incidence of catheter-related infections?"

Citation/Funding	Sample/Research Design	Independent Variable/ Intervention	Dependent Variable/ Outcome	Significant Results	Limitations/ Gaps	Generalizability	Level of Evidence
Citation: Pratt RJ, Pellowe CM, Wilson JA, et al. Epic2 national evidence-based guidelines for preventing health care–associated infections in NHS hospitals in England. J Hosp Infect 2007;665(Suppl):S1–64 Funding: British government	Sample: Development team a nurse-led multi-professional team of researchers and specialist clinicians Research design: guideline	N/A	Outcome: infection associated with central venous catheters	1) Decontaminate the skin site with a single patient use application of alcoholic chlorhexidine gluconate solution (preferably 2% chlorhexidine gluconate in 70% isopropyl alcohol) before the insertion of a central venous access device. (Class A recommendation: a systematic review of randomized controlled trials or a body of evidence that consists principally of studies rated as 1+, is directly applicable to the target population, and demonstrates overall consistency of results)	Guideline recommendations not tested, but audit criteria identified	Yes, except to children less than 1 year of age	Level I

Citation: Morgan LM, Thomas DJ. Implementing evidence-based nursing practice in the pediatric intensive care unit. J Infusion Nurs 2007;30(2): 105–12 Funding: no source identified	Sample: PICU staff at major pediatric hospital Research design: descriptive study	N/A	Outcome: incidence of catheter-related bloodstream infections in children	1) Mean rate decrease to 3.0 per 1000 CVC days (2006) from 5.2 per 1000 catheter days (2005) with CVC practice bundle and monitoring performance, including skin antisepsis at catheter insertion site with 2% chlorhexidine	Statistical analysis methods, power calculations, and variables not clearly described	Yes	Level VI

2) Use a single patient use application of alcoholic povidone-iodine solution for patients with a history of chlorhexidine sensitivity. Allow the antiseptic to dry before inserting the central venous access device. (Class D/GPP recommendation: a recommendation for best practice based on the experience of the guideline development group)

(continued on next page)

Table 3
(continued)

Citation/Funding	Sample/Research Design	Independent Variable/ Intervention	Dependent Variable/ Outcome	Significant Results	Limitations/ Gaps	Generalizability	Level of Evidence
Citation: Infusion Nurses Society. Infusion nursing standards of practice. J Infusion Nurs 2006; 29(1 Suppl): S1–92 Funding: no source identified	Sample: Development team a committee of RN experts Research design: guideline	N/A	Outcome: infusion nursing practice criteria for infection control and safety compliance of access site preparation	1) Antiseptic solutions that should be used include alcohol, chlorhexidine gluconate, povidone-iodine, and tincture of iodine, as single agents or in combination. Formulations containing a combination of alcohol and chlorhexidine gluconate or povidone-iodine are preferred. 2) Use of chlorhexidine gluconate in infants weighing <1000 g has associated with contact dermatitis and should be used with caution in this patient population. 3) For neonates, isopropyl alcohol or products containing isopropyl alcohol are	Recommendations not explicit or tagged by level of evidence. Development strategy not discussed. Key stakeholders and guideline developers unknown. Unknown if guideline subjected to peer-review and testing.	Yes	Level II

Citation/Funding	Sample	Intervention	Outcome	Findings	Comments		Level
Citation: Lee OK, Johnston L. (2005). A systematic review for effective management of central venous catheters and catheter sites in acute care pediatric patients. Worldviews on Evidence Based Nursing 2005;2(1):4–13. Funding: no source identified	Sample: Randomized and nonrandomized controlled trials investigating catheter management strategies in prevention of CVC complications in hospitalized children 0–18 years Research design: systematic review	Intervention: type of skin preparations/ antiseptic/ antimicrobial ointment	Outcome: catheter-related bloodstream infections in pediatric hospitalized patients	not recommended for access site preparation. Povidone-iodine or chlorhexidine gluconate solution is recommended but requires complete removal after the preparatory procedure with sterile water or sterile 0.9% sodium chloride (USP) to prevent product absorption. 1) CVC sites prepped and cleansed daily with chlorhexidine gluconate versus povidone-iodine solutions showed no significant differences in catheter-related bacteremia overall. Subgroup analysis of patients <12 months old showed higher rate of bacteremia in povidone-iodine group versus chlorhexidine gluconate group, but was not statistically significant.	Meta-analysis of the study results not feasible due to differences in intervention and outcome measures. Statistical power calculations not done on individual study. Variable dressing techniques confounded results of individual study.	Yes	Level I

(continued on next page)

Table 3
(continued)

Citation/Funding	Sample/Research Design	Independent Variable/ Intervention	Dependent Variable/ Outcome	Significant Results	Limitations/ Gaps	Generalizability	Level of Evidence
Citation: O'Grady NP, Alexander M, Dellinger EP, et al. (2002). Guidelines for the prevention of intravascular catheter-related infections. Pediatrics 2002;110(5):1-24. Funding: US government	Sample: Development team a multidisciplinary team of medicine and nursing Research design: guideline	N/A	Outcome: intravascular catheter-related bloodstream infections	1) Disinfect clean skin with an appropriate antiseptic before catheter insertion and during dressing changes. Although a 2% chlorhexidine-based preparation is preferred, tincture of iodine, an iodophor, or 70% alcohol can be used. (Category IA recommendation: strongly recommended for implementation and strongly supported by well-designed experimental, clinical, or epidemiologic studies) 2) No recommendation can be made for the use of chlorhexidine in infants aged 2 months. (Unresolvedissue: no recommendation; practices for which insufficient evidence or no consensus regarding efficacy exist)	Development strategy and process to identify, select, and combine evidence was not described. Guideline recommendations not tested.	Yes	Level II

Abbreviations: CVC, central venous catheter; GPP, good practice point.
Courtesy of Alyce A. Schultz, PhD, RN, FAAN, Chandler, AZ.

of synthesizing research studies is to determine whether the strength of the evidence supports a change in practice."[1] At this phase of the process, the steps of evidence-based practice were used to guide the literature search, collection of the best evidence, and critical appraisal. An example of the evidence synthesis relevant to a policy or procedure is consideration of the clinical question for central venous catheters.

The PICO question identified was "Among pediatric hospitalized patients requiring a central venous catheter, does use of chlorhexidine gluconate scrub versus Betadine and alcohol scrub decrease the incidence of catheter-related infections?" Employing multiple search databases, three guidelines, one systematic review, and one descriptive study were collected. Because only studies can be appraised, the published expert opinion was summarized but not appraised. The studies were appraised and leveled for quality using the rapid critical appraisal tools from Melnyk and Fineout-Overholt.[2] One systematic review (level I), three guidelines (levels I and II), and one descriptive study (level VI) were appraised and assigned a quality level using the system for levels of evidence (Table 2). The body of evidence, or synthesis of all the studies collectively, was graded for quality, quantity, and consistency of the results using an adapted system (Box 2).[9] The grade for this body of evidence on chlorhexidine gluconate was grade B, that is, consistent findings from evidence levels II, III, IV, or V. A recommendation was made in support of continuing the practice of using chlorhexidine gluconate as an antiseptic agent in preventing catheter-related infections in pediatric patients undergoing insertion of a central venous catheter (Table 3).

The NPC, after viewing a demonstration, adopted the developed process that integrated leveled and graded evidence in conjunction with an online pediatric procedure manual into P&Ps. For members of the NPC to disseminate an educational plan and maintain the practice change, the evidence-based practice mentors conducted education sessions for council members. The education provided served as a plan for council members in collaboration with the educator group to further develop into a process for educating all staff regarding evidence-based P&Ps. Outcomes to be addressed are the effects of evidence-based P&Ps on patient safety, cost, length of stay, nurse work time, and flow.

INTEGRATE AND MAINTAIN

Outcomes of the process for integrating evidence into P&Ps consisted of development of an evidence-based P&P template, completion of 32 P&Ps that were evidence based, education provided to the NPC and unit educators group, and development of a plan to educate the entire nursing staff about the integration of evidence into P&Ps. The process outcome of a template to guide incorporation of evidence into P&Ps was approached with the goal of enhancing the safe provision of patient care. An additional outcome from the process included the completion of 32 P&Ps that were evidence based by mentors in collaboration with experts in the content area. The P&Ps, once completed, were submitted to the NPC to approve and disseminate to health care staff within the organization.

This dissemination will aid in the integration and maintenance of the practice change related to evidence-based P&Ps. Communication of the recommended change to stakeholders, including nurses at the point-of-care, will continue to occur through educational endeavors by the nurse educators in the form of education sessions, Power Point presentations on unit online sites, and group e-mails. Monitoring of the process and evaluation of outcomes will continue within the organization through follow-up of NPC members.

SUMMARY

The process of developing P&Ps that are based on evidence involves multiple steps performed by experts in both evidence-based practice and content areas. P&Ps based on evidence can support consistency in nursing practice. Consistency can promote safety in the care of children and families, supporting the strategic plan of the organization and the national health care agenda of safety and promotion of evidence-based decision making at the point-of-care.

REFERENCES

1. Rosswurm MA, Larrabee JH. A model for change to evidence-based practice. Image J Nurs Sch 1999;31(4):317-22.
2. Melnyk BM, Fineout-Overholt E. Evidence-based practice in nursing & healthcare: a guide to best practice. Philadelphia: Lippincott Williams & Wilkins; 2005.
3. Finkelman A, Kenner C, Teaching IOM. Implications of the Institute of Medicine reports for nursing education. Silver Spring (MD): American Nurses Association; 2007.
4. The Joint Commission. 2008 National Patient Safety Goals. May 28, 2008.
5. Dawes M. On the need for evidence-based general and family practice. Evid Based Med 1996;1:68-9.
6. Heater B, Becker A, Olson R. Nursing interventions and patient outcomes: a meta-analysis of studies. Nurs Res 1988;37:303 7.
7. Goode CJ, Tanaka DJ, Krugman M, et al. Outcomes from the use of an evidence-based practice guideline. Nurs Econ 2000;18(4):202-7.
8. Sicola V, Chesley DA. Development of the Texas Textbook Evaluation Tool (T-TET). Nurse Educ 1999;24(2):23-8.
9. Schiffer CA, Anderson K, Bennett C, et al. ASCO special article. Platelet transfusion for patients with cancer: clinical practice guidelines of the American Society of Clinical Oncology. J Clin Oncol 2001;19(5):1519-38.

Staff Nurses Creating Safe Passage with Evidence-Based Practice

Dora Bradley, PhD, RN-BC[a],*, John F. Dixon, MSN, RN, CNA, BC[b]

KEYWORDS

- Evidence-based practice • Professional practice models
- PARIHS • Transformational leadership • Synergy

Patient safety is one of the most critical issues for health care today.[1–5] The escalating need to decrease preventable complications serves as a significant catalyst to identify and use evidence-based practice (EBP) at the bedside. Decreasing preventable complications requires a synergistic relationship between the nurses at the bedside and nursing leadership. By virtue of their place relative to the patient, nurses are positioned to prevent errors and poor care decisions and also to assume a leadership role in advancing the use of evidence to promote safety and quality care.[1,2,6] Further, nursing leaders must be able to provide a unified perspective of nursing's contribution by highlighting the linkages among the practice environment, evidence-based nursing practice, quality of patient care, and outcomes.[1,7] At Baylor Health Care System (BHCS) the Professional Nursing Practice Model (PNPM) is used in conjunction with the Promoting Action on Research Implementation in Health Services (PARIHS) framework[8] to develop and implement critical strategies that have increased significantly the use of EBP to improve nursing practice and to promote "safe passage," the optimal outcome of nursing.[9]

The urgency of employing EBP at the bedside has never been greater. By putting into operation the PARIHS concepts of evidence, facilitation, and context together with the BHCS PNPM model, BHCS has created a number of structures and processes necessary for engaging nurses in EBP activities that promote safe passage for patients. This article presents an overview of the concepts and the specific structures and processes used to increase the use of EBP and improve patient safety.

---

[a] Nursing Professional Development, Baylor Health Care System, Corporate Office of Chief Nursing Officer, 2001 Bryan Tower, Suite 600, Dallas, TX 75201, USA
[b] BUMC Center for Nursing Education and Research, Baylor University Medical Center, 3500 Gaston Avenue, Dallas, TX 75246, USA
* Corresponding author.
E-mail address: dora.bradley@baylorhealth.edu (D. Bradley).

Nurs Clin N Am 44 (2009) 71–81
doi:10.1016/j.cnur.2008.10.002   nursing.theclinics.com

CREATING URGENCY FOR EVIDENCE-BASED PRACTICE

In recent months, the Centers for Medicare and Medicaid Services (CMS) has promoted a culture of progressively greater provider accountability.[4] Building on the Institute of Medicine report, To Err is Human: Building a Safer Health System,[3] the CMS created a plan that will deny extra reimbursement for hospitals if a patient develops a preventable complication during the hospitalization. Currently the plan to be implemented in October 2008 includes eight non-reimbursable conditions, and that number may increase significantly by 2010. These reimbursement issues, coupled with the increasing public awareness of errors and avoidable hospital complications occurring throughout the nation, have created a new sense of urgency for hospitals to find ways to prevent complications. Consequently, hospitals are being compelled to allocate significant resources to identifying and implementing strategies and processes that will decrease the occurrence of avoidable complications. Even though complications are everyone's concern, it makes sense to focus on supporting nursing efforts, because nurses typically are closest to the patient and many of these non-reimbursable conditions (eg, pressure ulcers, catheter-associated urinary tract infections, and falls with injuries) are nurse-sensitive outcomes.[10] Therefore, it is imperative that nurses be able to employ the most effective actions to prevent these outcomes.

In the recent Agency for Healthcare Research and Quality (AHRQ) publication, Patient Safety and Quality: An Evidence-Based Handbook for Nurses,[1] the Director of AHRQ and the President and Chief Executive Officer of the Hobert Wood Johnson Foundation stated that "high-quality health care can be achieved through the use of evidence and an enabled and empowered nursing workforce."[1] Consequently, the need to empower and support nurses to identify and use EBP related to patient safety has a significant likelihood of resulting in better patient outcomes and also in a substantial return on investment.

So what does nursing need to do? Nursing generally has stressed the importance of patient safety but has not always been able to articulate the nursing practices that are designed to prevent harm and create safe passage of patients.[1] Florence Nightingale set the stage for using evidence and data to make decisions about patient safety and prevention. After Nightingale, however, nursing's knowledge development seems to have been based more on tradition than on evidence. Now there is increasing evidence that some tradition-based practices may not promote the type of outcomes they once were thought to do.[11,12] Conversely, there is substantial verification that specific evidence-based nursing practices can decrease patient complications and adverse events.[1,11] Therefore, if nursing's identification and use of EBP can decrease complications, it is imperative that hospitals and nursing leadership create structures and processes to promote the development and implementation of evidence-based nursing practices. Not implementing EBP could be considered unethical.

FACTORS INFLUENCING THE IMPLEMENTATION OF EVIDENCE-BASED PRACTICE

Because of external forces, hospitals will need to make aggressive changes in current practices to ensure that patients do not experience avoidable complications during hospitalization. To meet fiscal goals, organizations must look at the growing evidence demonstrating the significant link between the identification and implementation of EBP and improved patient outcomes.[1,4,5] Therefore, the allocation of resources for the creation of effective structures and processes to support EBP will be critical both to patient safety and to the fiscal goals of the organization. To create a supportive environment, organizations need to identify and develop strategies that have the highest potential of influencing the successful implementation of EBP. The PARIHS

framework[8,13] purports that successful implementation of EBP at the bedside relates directly to the functions of evidence, facilitation, and context. The function of evidence reflects knowledge sources, which include research, clinical experience, patient experience, and local data and information. Facilitation is a function that relates to assisting with the implementation of EBP and is operationalized in the role, skills, and attributes of the facilitator. Context function represents the culture, leadership, and evaluation processes in the environment where practice changes need to occur.

Using the PARIHS framework as a guide to decrease complications and improve quality, nursing leaders must transform infrastructures in the work environment to integrate EBP into bedside nursing practice. Successful implementation of EBP at the bedside requires nurses to have ready access to meaningful information and data, specifically library access, patient preference information, and meaningful quality data. In addition, allocation of funds and other resources is critical to support the development of EBP expertise and credible practice changes. To create an "EBP context," transformational nursing leaders must work with staff to create a vision for EBP at the bedside, create opportunities for nurses to question practice, promote risk-taking, and value questioning of practice.[14] In addition, strategies that support development and create opportunities for recognition are critical to the effort. Some examples are advancement programs that promote the use of EBP, nurse councils in which nurses make decisions to change practices based on evidence, and methods to create ongoing feedback. By operationalizing the functions of the PARIHS framework in conjunction with defined practice models, nursing leaders have the means to integrate EBP at the bedside and improve patient outcomes.

BAYLOR HEALTH CARE SYSTEM PROFESSIONAL NURSING PRACTICE MODEL

The system's chief nursing officers adopted the BHCS PNPM in 2005 (**Fig. 1**). At its core is the American Association of Critical-Care Nurses (AACN) Synergy Model for Patient Care.[9] The Synergy Model is based on studies of practice and clearly articulates the importance of the linkage between nurse competencies and patient needs, regardless of practice specialty. The premise of the Synergy Model is that when patient needs are matched to nurse competencies, synergistic nursing practice results in safe passage defined as "an optimal outcome of nursing."[9] BHCS has expanded on the original definition by describing safe passage as "an optimal outcome of nursing. Nurses promote safe passage for their patients by using knowledge of patient needs and the health care environment to assist them to transition through the health care encounter without any preventable complications or delay."[15]

The patient's need for safe passage is a catalyst for EBP. Within the Synergy Model,[9] there are eight areas of patient need and eight nurse competencies. The nurse competencies have operational definitions that are defined further on a continuum from baseline competence to expert level. The areas of patient need reflect a holistic assessment going beyond the physiologic system approach of the traditional medical model. This holistic approach includes distinctive areas best addressed by the unique contributions of nursing practice through interventions such as facilitation of learning, responsiveness to diversity, and creation of supportive and healing therapeutic environments. The model also reflects the importance of nurses being autonomous, having the authority to change or modify their practice, and the expectation that nurses take accountability for their actions and the resulting outcomes. In addition, the model recognizes that nursing practice does not occur within a vacuum but rather interacts with a complex work environment that surrounds it. To address this phenomenon, BHCS incorporated the AACN's Healthy Work Environment Standards[16] as part of

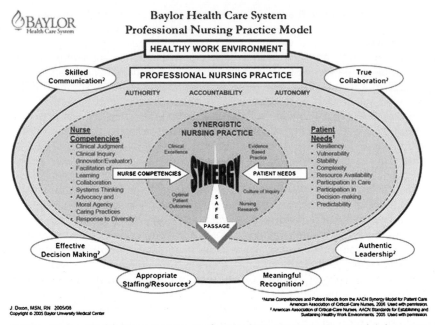

Fig. 1. The Baylor Health Care System Professional Nursing Practice Model (*Courtesy of Baylor Health Care System, Dallas, TX; with permission.*)

the PNPM. To promote synergistic nursing practice, the immediate work environment must be one that supports the development of a culture of inquiry, expects clinical excellence and optimal patient outcomes, and fosters nursing research and EBP. The PNPM provides a framework for professional practice and clearly articulates important concepts and linkages suitable for EBP projects and research.

ENGAGING NURSES IN EVIDENCE-BASED PRACTICE TO PROMOTE SAFE PASSAGE

BHCS has used specific strategies to engage nurses in EBP while assisting them to promote safe passage of their patients. By applying the PARIHS functions of evidence, facilitation, and context to the PNPM concepts, BHCS has been able to operationalize a number of the successful strategies that link EBP, nursing practice, and patient outcomes.

Evidence

Increasing the staff nurses' access to evidence, including research, data, and benchmarking information, was the first essential strategy. The BHCS library provides outstanding services and resources in support of Baylor's evidence-based nursing practice, nursing research efforts, and nursing practice specialties. The library's online resources, including more than 250 full-text nursing journals, dozens of full-text nursing books, and a wide variety of literature databases, are available from any computer in the BHCS network. The librarians are available for customized classes, one-on-one training sessions, researching tough questions, and performing literature searches—all free of charge to any nurse. These resources have been used to explore and support changes in both administrative and clinical practices.

With increased awareness of EBP and the implementation of Baylor's professional nursing advancement program ("Achieving Synergy in Practice through Impact, Relationships, and Evidence," ASPIRE), Cumulative Index of Nursing and Allied Health Literature (CINAHL) searches increased by 17% from 2006 to 2007 (2007 = 6806), CINAHL sessions increased by 26% (2007 = 2140), and access to nursing journals increased by 12% (2007 = 3752).

To understand patient preferences as a source of evidence, nurses have used patient satisfaction data and unit interviews. A number of nurses have conducted focus groups to identify patients' preferences for various aspects of care and learning. The neonatal ICU (NICU) nurses completed an EBP project to determine the best practices for discharge-to-home education of parents with potentially fragile infants. Over the years, the NICU nurses had compiled a very comprehensive discharge education program. They were challenged to identify whether their current practices were truly evidenced based. They reviewed the literature and found some important differences in their approach, especially for the younger parents. To identify patient/family preferences, they sought information from families attending the annual NICU day. They discovered that much of the material they were providing to families was based on what the staff thought was critical, not on what the family really needed. Consequently, the NICU made significant evidence-based changes to the discharge education program.

As in many other large facilities, access to meaningful local data and reports has been somewhat difficult at times. BHCS leadership, however, is committed to transparency, and therefore nursing leadership, staff, and others have spent considerable time creating staff nurse access to unit-based data. Now, unit data are available with trends and comparisons to other like units, the hospital, the system, and national benchmarks, when available. This effort has yielded a number of EBP projects related to falls, urinary tract infections, ventilator-acquired pneumonia, and pressure ulcers. These projects have resulted in decreased complication rates and have provided the foundation for changes in practice on individual units and frequently across units and multiple facilities within the BHCS.

Facilitation

To facilitate the ongoing growth of EBP, the goal has been to assist managers and staff in gaining the skills and knowledge necessary to recognize the need for change and the steps they need to take to get the desired outcomes. Consequently, a Research and EBP series was developed. In 2007 and 2008, experts in the areas of EBP and research were invited to provide education and consultation at various venues throughout BHCS. Some of the topics presented included creating a culture of inquiry, determining a clinically significant problem and writing the clinical question, evaluating and critiquing primary studies and systematic reviews, and linking EBP and research to patient outcomes. Groups and individuals also participated in private consultations to refine their projects. The result was a significant increase in both EBP projects and research studies. Most of the projects focused on improving patient outcomes and decreasing complications conceptualized within the PNPM.

The Evidence-Based Nursing Practice and Nursing Research Council was created to facilitate practice changes and the ongoing development of EBP and research skills. The charge of this council is to "develop and validate knowledge to advance the science and practice of nursing through the promotion and support of Evidence-Based Nursing Practice (EBNP) and Nursing Research at Baylor." The Council is responsible for (1) providing a setting to evaluate nursing practice against best practices and current evidence; (2) recommending the implementation of specific nursing protocols, procedures, and guidelines to promote best practice; (3) improving patient care, safety, and outcomes; and (4) serving as a clearinghouse for evidence-based nursing practice and nursing research projects. Membership is primarily staff nurses from all nursing specialties but also includes representatives from education, management, and advanced practice. This council makes evidence-based recommendations for practice and policy changes to the Staff Nurse Advisory Council.

To provide a consistent approach, several key structures have been adopted to facilitate EBP. The Iowa model serves as a guideline for identifying and processing triggers for potential EBP projects.[17] Questions are formulated using the PICO format, but with a slight modification. An "S" has been added to PICO to represent "Safe Passage and Synergy," thus ensuring that the question links to the BHCS PNPM (**Fig. 2**). The strength of the evidence is graded using the Stetler level of evidence table.[18]

Two practice changes that the EBP council facilitated are practices in the insertion and routine care of urinary catheters and eliminating saline instillation before suctioning into endotracheal tubes. Both these practices tie directly to EBP and Safe Passage: evidence is being used to direct practice to minimize the risk of preventable complications and delays so that the patient can continue to move along the health care continuum.

Context

The focus on decreasing patient complications and the use of EBP has been a "strategic direction" for the entire BHCS during the last few years. There has been a major effort to cascade these strategic goals for EBP and patient safety in a meaningful way to the unit level. Because of this focus on EBP and safety, resources are allocated to this initiative for all patient care disciplines. Within the nursing departments, a number of hospitals in the Baylor Healthcare System are seeking Magnet designation, providing tremendous contextual support for EBP initiatives.[7]

Recent revisions in nursing job descriptions include expectations for the staff nurse in the area of clinical inquiry. Specifically the staff nurse is expected (1) to question and evaluate practice and provide EBP; (2) to create practice changes through research use and experiential learning; and (3) to support the implementation of changes and EBP. These expectations are reflected in the regular performance appraisals.

Other contextual factors include EBP as a focus during nursing orientation and new graduate internships. Nursing leaders promote the expectation for use of evidence in practice through an introduction in nursing orientation. There is a strong focus on EBP in all the internship programs. The recent revision of internship goals and outcomes reflects the practice model and includes a significant focus on EBP (**Table 1**) Learning content is included in both didactic and clinical practice. Unit or service-line educators evaluate the achievement of outcomes on the unit through the completion of specific learning activities. The preceptor, clinical nurse specialist, and/or unit educator keys in on a specific "why is it done this way" question asked by the nurse intern. The nurse intern is expected to use the unit computer to access articles related to the practice. to review the data and to create a method for sharing findings with other nurses on the unit. The nurse educator and/or clinical nurse specialist validates the results.

LINKING NURSING EVIDENCE AND PATIENT OUTCOMES

BHCS has created a number of strategies to identify opportunities support EBP. One of the most important programs is the professional nursing advancement program, ASPIRE. ASPIRE was created in 2005 to recognize the registered nurse's unique contributions to patient outcomes. The program defines nursing practice as the integration of

PICO-S

Asking Your Burning Clinical Question

Whether doing an evidence-based practice review or conducting a nursing research study, you start with a question. If your question is focused and well-thought out then your efforts will be easier because you will have a clear direction of how to proceed.

Burning Clinical Questions can arise from a number of triggers such as:
...**data** (e.g., quality, risk management, financial, benchmarks) ...a **clinical problem or process** you identify
...**standards and guidelines** from national nursing organizations ...a recently **published article**
To help create a focused, well-thought out question, we are using the PICO-S format. The better you craft your question, the clearer it is to determine specific steps you need to take.

P Patient or Problem	I Intervention	C Comparison	O Outcome(s)	S Synergy & Safe Passage
• Define who will make up this population, addressing who will be included and, if appropriate, who will be excluded • Define what the problem is	• Define the intervention	• Define who/what will be used as the comparison, could be another group like a control group or themselves if doing a pre- then post- test with the same group	• Define what outcomes are to be measured and how these will be measured	• Identify which patient needs and/or nurse competencies align with this initiative • Think about how this project will contribute to Safe Passage
Example				
Patients to be fed using a nasogastric tube	Verification of nasogastric tube placement	Current practice versus the evidence	Correct placement of nasogastric tube.	Safe Passage - Feeding delivered into the gut. Patient Need – *Vulnerability* – at risk for inappropriate placement Nurse Competency – *Clinical Judgment* – refined assessment

Fig. 2. Baylor Health Care System PICO-S question template. (*Courtesy of* Baylor Health Care System, Dallas, TX; with permission.)

knowledge, skills, experience, and attitudes that, when linked to the patient needs and characteristics, creates a synergistic process that results in safe passage and optimal outcomes.

The program has three levels, colleague, mentor, and leader. The scope and level of outcomes differentiates the three levels. There are a number of components that must be completed. First are the required elements, which address experience, education, certification, EBP, learning opportunities, and nursing's unique contribution to outcomes. Many have used the required EBP activity as the overall direction and support for the other activities of their plans. **Table 2** shows the requirements and expected evidence for EBP at each level.

There are four areas of development: clinical practice, leadership, education, and best practices. Each of these areas is linked specifically to one or more of the eight

Table 1
Baylor health care system competency expectations for nursing interns

Nurse Competency	Key Criteria/Interactions to Identify	Learning Content	Outcomes
Clinical inquiry (innovator/evaluator)	Incorporates evidence-based practice/best practices into daily care	Exposure to evidence-based practice/research	By completion of orientation, the interns will identify questions related to practice and be able to access research/ best practices in their field of expertise. They will do this by:
	Accesses unit QI data/infection rates and explains how best practices contribute to patient safety	Resources to access	Recognizing the evidence based/best practices used in their specialty areas
	Questions practice and accesses online resources to identify research findings	ASPIRE	Questioning why practices in health care are "done this way"
		Professional organizations	Accessing the online Health Sciences Library and locating research articles related to their practice questions
		Educational offerings	Recognizing systems in place to improve practice (nursing councils)
		Certification	

Courtesy of Baylor Health Care System, Dallas, TX; with permission.

nurse competencies of the Synergy model. The nurse chooses to develop one activity from each area. In addition, two optional activities can be used to replace some of the specialty development areas. For example, the nurse can conduct a formal research study approved by the institutional review board in which the nurse is the principal investigator or can write and submit a formal manuscript for publication in a national nursing journal.

The outcomes of the ASPIRE program have been outstanding. Through clinical narratives, nurses have documented the ways their intentional nursing actions have had a positive impact on patient or unit outcomes. As would be expected in a large academic medical center, medical practice is predominant. The EBP review has required staff to focus on nursing practice's unique contribution to patient care. Some of the initial plans identified medical practices or procedures as the EBP focus, but through mentoring and coaching, staff members were able to translate these foci into nursing practice. For instance, one nurse wanted to conduct an EBP review on anesthesia given

Table 2 ASPIRE: three levels of requirements for evidence-based nursing practice		
Colleague	**Mentor**	**Leader**
Assists with the identification of a patient or practice problem by gathering, analyzing baseline information, and presenting recommendations for considerations to Unit-based Partnership Council	Uses an evidence-based nursing practice review to create or validate a practice and formally presents findings to Unit-based Partnership Council	Implements and evaluates an evidence-based nursing practice change and formally presents to housewide Best Care Partnership Council
Evidence: Overview of baseline information, collection method, analysis and recommendations presented to partnership council; minutes from council	Evidence: Provide evidence-based indicators used to evaluate nursing practice and the results; minutes of partnership council	Evidence: Description of the process used to implement change and the resulting outcomes; minutes of partnership council

Modified from Baylor Health Care System; with permission.

during circumcision. Anesthesia is not determined or administered by nurses. Discussion with the nurse revealed that her interest lay predominantly pain management for infants undergoing circumcision. With help in crafting her question and redirecting her energies, she was able to identify nursing practices to support effective pain management of infants undergoing this procedure.

Many of the EBP projects addressed in the ASPIRE projects are based on situations that bedside practitioners encounter on a routine basis. Some of these practices include difficult intravenous starts in cold procedural areas, ineffective assessment of the risk for falls or pressure ulcers, inadequate patient and family teaching practices, and many others. Consistent with this culture of inquiry, these individuals now ask why a practice is followed and what evidence supports current practices. As a result, nurses are thinking about the evidence that supports daily nursing practices. In addition, the process of participating in ASPIRE is helping strengthen further the EBP knowledge and skills of staff, advancing the culture of inquiry.

Positive Patient Outcomes

Two of the many examples of the work nurses have done are described here in more depth. One nurse decided to look at the safe passage of patients who had a prior history of lymphadenectomy or mastectomy and who were undergoing some other type of surgical procedure. The vulnerability she identified was that these patients could not participate in their care or decision making when sedated; thus, they could not tell practitioners not to use their affected arm. From her own family members' experiences, she knew that this situation could create fear and anxiety. She decided that there had to be a better way inform all health care practitioners encountering the patient of the existence of these affected extremities. From her efforts in examining communication and handoff practices in the literature and benchmarking with other hospitals, she initiated the pink bracelet pilot project. In the day surgery hospital, a pink armband was placed on the affected extremity of patients who had a known history of lymphadenectomy or mastectomy. The reaction from patients was so extremely positive that several asked to meet the nurse who had developed this program. After the pilot, one patient who returned for an additional day hospital procedure refused to go to the operating room until she had her pink bracelet. As a result, the pink bracelet identification project is being used system-wide, and this nurse now is the principal investigator on a nursing research study to measure the bracelet's effect in reducing anxiety and fear.

The second example of positive change in practice based on inquiry and evidence occurred in one of the ICUs. A nurse identified that a coordinated plan for initiating weaning of patients from ventilators was lacking, thus making the patients vulnerable for potential complications and delays. She began her exploration by reviewing the literature, where she found a reliable and valid method for assessing readiness to wean from the ventilator.[19] Through her research, she learned that most practitioners focus on a only few primary pulmonary factors. Using this baseline knowledge assessment, she instituted a series of learning interventions. Postassessments demonstrated a significant increase in staff's knowledge of pulmonary and nonpulmonary factors that affect readiness to wean. Additionally, she applied the weaning-readiness screening tool and identified a number of patients who met the readiness criteria but had not been provided with a weaning trial. These missed opportunities resulted in delay in weaning and extubation, an outcome contrary to safe passage. The results of her nursing intervention have been shared with the critical care service line, and plans now are underway to consider routine implementation of the screening tool for all mechanically ventilated patients.

In both these ASPIRE projects, the nurses identified patients who were vulnerable and had a high potential for complications or adverse reactions. They responded with EBP initiatives and collected measurable data on nursing's unique contribution to outcomes and safe passage. A recent evaluation of the ASPIRE program found that nurses across the system identified evidence-based nursing practice as an essential element of current nursing practice and thought it should continue to be a required element.

SUMMARY

Focusing on the development of evidence, context, and facilitation functions within the practice environment is likely to assist nurses in identifying and implementing EBP. In addition, by demonstrating their ability to decrease complications and improve patient outcomes, nurses can demonstrate their significant contribution to patient care and organizational stewardship. The true challenge, however, still may be in getting nurses to realize that EBP can empower them to demonstrate the significant impact on outcomes and the safe passage of their patients.

REFERENCES

1. Hughes RG. Patient safety and quality: an evidence-based handbook for nurses. Rockville (MD): Agency for Healthcare Research and Quality; 2008. AHRQ Publication No. 08-0043.
2. Clancy CM, Farquhar MB, sharp BA. Patient safety in nursing practice. J Nurs Care Qual 2005;20(3):193–7.
3. Kohn LT, Corrigan JM, Donaldson MS, editors. To err is human: building a safer health care system. Washington, DC: National Academy Press, Institute of Medicine; 1999.

4. Centers for Medicare and Medicaid Services Office of Public Affairs. CMS proposes to expand quality program for hospital inpatient service in FY 2009 [April 14, 2008 press release]. Available at: http://www.cms.hhs.gov/apps/media/press/release. asp?Counter=3041&;intNumPerPage=10&checkDate=1&checkKey=2&srchType =3&numDays=90&srchOpt=0&srchData=quality&keywordType=All&chkNews Type=1%2C+2%2C+3%2C+4%2C+5&intPage=&showAll=1&pYear=&year= 0&desc=&cboOrder=date. Accessed May18, 2008.
5. Leape LL. Advances in patient safety: from research to implementation. In: Implementation issues, Vol 3. Rockville (MD): Agency for Healthcare Research and Quality; 2005. AHRQ Publication No. 05-0021-3.
6. Institute of Medicine. Keeping patients safe: transforming the work environment of nurses. Washington, DC: National Academies Press; 2004.
7. American Nurses Credentialing Center. Overview of ANCC magnet recognition program new model [brochure]. Available at: http://www.nursecredentialing.org/ model/MagnetModel.pdf. Accessed June 19, 2008.
8. Rycroft-Malone J. The PARIHS framework: a framework for guiding the implementation of evidence-based practice. J Nurs Care Qual 2004;19(4):297–304.
9. Curley MA. Patient–nurse synergy: optimizing patients' outcomes. Am J Crit Care 1998;7(1):64–72.
10. National Quality Forum. Nation consensus standards for nursing-sensitive care: an initial performance measure set. Washington, DC: National Quality Forum; 2004.
11. Rauen CA, Chulay M, Bridges E, et al. Seven evidence-based practice habits: putting some sacred cows out to pasture. Crit Care Nurse 2008;28(2):98–124.
12. Nursing staffing and patient outcomes in the inpatient setting: report. Washington, DC: American Nurses Association; 2000.
13. Cummings GC, Estabrooks CA, Midodzi WK, et al. Influence of organizational characteristics and context on research utilization. Nurse Res 2007;56(4S): S24–39.
14. McCormack B, Kitson A, Harvey G, et al. Getting evidence into practice: the meaning of "context". J Adv Nurs 2002;38(1):94–104.
15. Dixon JF, Bradley D. Implementing a synergistic professional nursing practice model. In: Curley AQ, editor. Synergy: the unique relationship between nurses and patients. Indianapolis (IN): Sigma Theta Tau; 2007. p. 119–28.
16. AACN standards for establishing and sustaining health work environments: a journey to excellence. Aliso Viejo (CA): Amreican Association of Critical-Care Nurses; 2005.
17. Titler MG, Kleiber C, Steelman VJ, et al. The Iowa model of evidence-based practice to promote quality care. Crit Care Nurs Clin North Am 2001;13(4):497–509.
18. Stetler C. Updating the Stetler model of research utilization to facilitate evidence-based practice. Nurs Outlook 2001;49(6):272–8.
19. Burns SM, Earven S, Fisher C, et al. Implementation of an institutional program to improve clinical and financial outcomes of mechanically ventilated patients: one-year outcomes and lessons learned. Crit Care Med 2003;31(12):2752–63.

A Nursing Quality Program Driven by Evidence-Based Practice

Jacqueline J. Anderson, MSN, RN[a,b],
Marilyn Mokracek, MSN, RN, CCRN, NE-BC[c,d],
Cheryl N. Lindy, PhD, RN-BC, NEA-BC[e,*]

KEYWORDS

• Nursing quality • Best practice • Evidence-based practice

St. Luke's Episcopal Hospital in Houston established a best-practice council as a vehicle for identifying critical issues at the hospital and focusing on improving outcomes. Committed to convene, charge, and direct small interdisciplinary work teams, this Best Practice Council replaced the traditional nursing-quality council. The traditional nursing-quality program had focused on nursing documentation compliance rather than on quality improvement. Under that program, the nursing staff completed monthly chart reviews and submitted the audits as part of the nursing service quality program. However, the unit manager rarely audited nursing documentation for compliance with organizational policies. The nursing staff was required to review nursing documentation and collect data on peers. Completion of the audits was a requirement to receive a "meets" score on the staff nurse annual performance evaluation. Therefore, each nurse manager was required to track the completion of the quality audits and follow up with those whose audits were incomplete. The program consumed an extensive amount of time of both nursing staff and unit management. The nursing staff

---

[a] Division of Nursing, Unit 82, The University of Texas MD Anderson Cancer Center, 1515 Holcombe Boulevard, Houston, TX 77030, USA
[b] Nursing Research, St. Luke's Episcopal Hospital, 6720 Bertner Avenue, MC4-278, Houston, TX 77030, USA
[c] Neurosciences Service, St. Luke's Episcopal Hospital, 6720 Bertner Avenue, MC4-278, Houston, TX 77030, USA
[d] Best Practice Council, St. Luke's Episcopal Hospital, 6720 Bertner Avenue, MC4-278, Houston, TX 77030, USA
[e] Nursing and Patient Education and Research, St. Luke's Episcopal Hospital, 6720 Bertner Avenue, MC4-278, Houston, TX 77030, USA
* Corresponding author. Nursing and Patient Education and Research, St. Luke's Episcopal Hospital, 6720 Bertner Avenue, MC4-278, Houston, TX 77030, USA.
E-mail address: 77030janderson@mdanderson.org (J.J. Anderson).

Nurs Clin N Am 44 (2009) 83–91
doi:10.1016/j.cnur.2008.10.012
0029-6465/08/$ – see front matter © 2009 Elsevier Inc. All rights reserved.

did not see value in the completion of the audits because rarely was any action taken to improve the outcome findings. The time-intensive tasks of auditing charts left no opportunity for staff to become involved in actual improvement projects.

Unit outcomes data were reported to the nursing directors and filtered to the nurse managers with assignments for developing action plans to correct variances in their department data. Quality scores determined by nursing audits were often inconsistent with outcomes data reported through other departments. The traditional program also resulted in several teams working on the same problem completely unaware that another department had already identified the problem and implemented a practice change.

The main purpose of the Best Practice Council was to investigate clinical outcomes variances and provide clinically relevant direction to enhance patient care. The aim of the council was to legislate and standardize practice change across the hospital based on evidence of best practice. The council developed mechanisms to share best practices and eliminate duplicate efforts.

BEST PRACTICE COUNCIL

The Best Practice Council consisted of nursing leaders and staff nurses committed to enhancing patient outcomes through evidence-based practice. The council established work teams based on areas identified for performance improvement. Team leaders were identified and interdisciplinary team membership was assigned from multiple units. Teams were given clearly defined goals and responsibilities with the requirement to provide a progress report at the monthly Best Practice Council meeting. Each team was charged with identifying the problem or opportunity for improvement through the development of a problem statement. Each team assessed current practice and outcomes data, reviewed the current research, and made recommendations for changes to policies and practice. Once the best practice was identified and tested within the organization's culture, the team made recommendations for evaluation to ensure continued success. The Best Practice Council reviewed and tracked each team's performance and made recommendations for organizational implementation of "best practice" for each specific topic. According to the original plan, once a team's goals were met, the team would be disbanded and new teams would be created.

The team leader was responsible for scheduling the team meetings, developing the agenda, and ensuring that minutes were recorded. The first meetings were dedicated to getting the team organized. The team leader reviewed the quality data with the team, clarified the problem or opportunity for improvement, and developed a list of available and potential resources that might be required. The team completed a review of the literature related to the clinical issue. Based on the results and the action required, the team developed measurable goals and a timeline for completion of the project.

ST. LUKE'S EVIDENCE BASED PRACTICE MODEL

The teams each used the St. Luke's Evidence Based Practice Model (**Fig. 1**) as a guide. Adopted by the hospital's Division of Nursing in 2006, the model was developed for research use in the mid-1990s by the hospital's nurse researcher and Nursing Research Council. The original model was based on the Iowa Model of Evidence Based Practice to Promote Quality Care.[1]

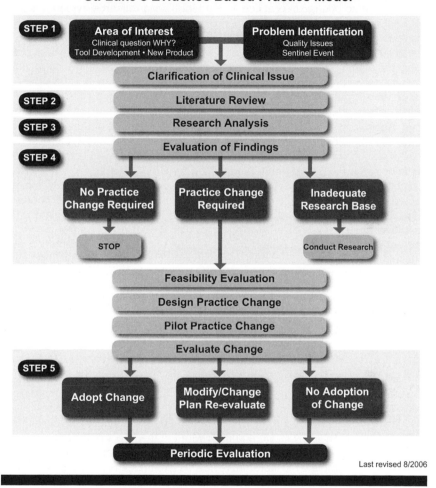

Fig. 1. St. Luke's Evidence Based Practice Model. (*Courtesy of* St. Luke's Episcopal Hospital, Houston, TX; with permission. Copyright © 2006, St. Luke's Episcopal Hospital.)

The model was updated in 2006 to favor an evidence-based practice approach. Melnyk and Fineout-Overholt,[2] in outlining the process for comparison, identified five key steps to the process of evidence-based practice:

1. Ask the burning question.
2. Collect the most relevant and best evidence.
3. Critically appraise the evidence.
4. Integrate the evidence with one's clinical expertise, patient preferences, and values in making a practice decision or change.
5. Evaluate the practice decision or change.[2]

These fives steps were highlighted in the model as shown in **Fig. 1**.

As a guide for each team, the St. Luke's Evidence Based Practice Model enumerates the steps that lead to each major decision that must be made. The first decision is reached after critical assessment of current practice and evaluation of relevant literature. Three outcomes are possible at this point. The first possible outcome is a recommendation that no change in practice is needed. If solid research evidence supports the current practice, then the decision is to make no changes. The second potential outcome is the finding that sufficient evidence supports making a change. The third potential outcome is the finding that evidence is insufficient to determine best practice and that the team needs to conduct further research to answer the question at hand.

When evidence supports change, the subsequent steps of the model lead the individual or team through the steps of designing and implementing that change. The final decision comes after completing a pilot and evaluating the impact of the practice change. Again, any of three outcomes are possible. The result of the pilot may demonstrate that the intended impact was not achieved and, for a variety of reasons, the change in practice may not be practical. The proposed change is then not adopted for the time being and the team returns to the literature to research alternative solutions. The second and rare outcome is that the practice change worked perfectly, exactly as expected, and is ready to be put into practice as a permanent and house-wide change. The third and more common outcome is that additional modifications are needed and another pilot called for. This step is repeated until the practice change consistently produces the required results and is ready for implementation across the hospital setting. This process mirrors the organizational quality improvement model and each team presents its results using the plan–do–check/study–act design.

USING OR IMPLEMENTING THE BEST PRACTICE MODEL

After the Best Practice Council completed the initial step of problem identification, each team was established based on quality outcome data that reflected potential areas for improvement. The director of nursing research was assigned to assist each team leader in getting the teams started. The director explained the evidence-based practice model to team members and described the steps each team needed to follow in working through the process. The first meeting was used to clarify the clinical issue and develop key search terms. At subsequent meetings, the relevant literature and a method for analysis were shared with the members of the team.

In critiquing literature and drawing conclusions, each team acted differently. Some teams elected to complete the literature review as a team. Others divided the literature and reviewed the studies as smaller groups within the team. Each team had a different experience with the literature. For example, the members assigned to the Pressure Ulcer Best Practice Team reviewed an abundance of literature from a number of different disciplines. In contrast, the Communication Hand-Off Best Practice Team found several studies related to team communication and emergency situations in other industries, but little evidence on communication between shifts or among departments within hospitals. The conclusions reached by each team after reviewing evidence and making comparisons to current practice are discussed below.

The Best Practice Council expected that each team would require 4 to 6 months to assess current practice and data results, review the current research and evidence related to the practice, and make recommendations for changes in policy and practice. Once the work of the current teams was completed, new teams for new target areas would be identified. The team members used the evidence-based practice model described above to focus concerns and questions, search for relevant evidence, and determine the applicability and feasibility of necessary changes. The first teams were assigned to study best practice in (1) preventing bloodstream infection (related to central lines); (2) preventing patient falls; (3) assessing and preventing pressure ulcers; and (4) ensuring good hand-off communication. The activities of the teams are described below.

Bloodstream Infection Prevention Best Practice Team

The Blood Stream Infection Prevention Best Practice Team focused on bloodstream infections related to the presence of central lines in the intensive care unit (ICU). In September 2006, when this team was formed, there were 11 ICUs in the institution. Five of the units ranked within the top 10th percentile in the National Nosocomial Infections Surveillance database, which provides the infection control benchmarks.[3] The remaining units were still well below the 50th percentile. An interdisciplinary team was formed with staff nurses, nurse managers, infection control practitioners, a critical care clinical nurse specialist, a nurse researcher, and an intravenous therapy nurse. Through use of the evidence-based practice model, the team conducted an extensive literature review, which was enhanced by the use of an annotated bibliography from the Institute for Healthcare Improvement[4] and of guidelines to prevent catheter-related infections from the Centers for Disease Control and Prevention.[5] Information from the literature was synthesized and compared with the current policy and procedures regarding insertion and care of central lines. The practices of the ICUs that ranked within the top 10th percentile were also evaluated for best practice. The team found that in comparing policy to best practice, only two minor revisions needed to be made. The policy was revised to include regular "dead end" cap changes and end the practice of placing a gauze over the insertion site underneath the clear dressing. The team also found a critical gap in the process of ensuring proper procedures: The bedside nurse was powerless to stop an insertion if any step in the proper process was omitted. To correct this problem, the team introduced a checklist to empower the nurse to assess and intervene if necessary.[6] Meanwhile, in reviewing practices in all of the hospitals's ICUs, the team found that the ICU with lowest infection rate used a sign to indicate the day the dressing needed to be changed. All of the hospital's ICUs came to adopt each of these changes—implementing the "dead-end" cap, ending the use of gauze over the insertion site, introducing a checklist, and posting signs calling for dressings to be changed. The bloodstream infection rates are reported monthly. The rate has improved and, with the exception of two units, remains well below the benchmark of the 50th percentile.

Fall Prevention Best Practice Team

The Fall Prevention Best Practice Team was assembled to identify innovative approaches to prevent falls. Team members included nursing staff and management, physical therapists, radiologists, clinical nurse specialists, and nursing researchers. A review of current practice revealed that fall risks were being assessed using the Hendrich II Fall Risk Assessment Tool,[7] which was completed every shift. The review also found that the rates of both falls and falls with injury were increasing. The interdisciplinary team determined that innovative strategies needed to be developed for patients identified at high risk of falling. A review of the literature initially revealed 131 research articles. After research criteria were limited to include only those articles from the past 3 years that focused on innovative interventions and that had scientific merit, 9 research studies were selected. These studies, all related to fall prevention, focused on (1) patient assessment,[8–11] (2) patients' needs for excessive toileting and effects of medications,[9,10] (3) staff, patient, and family education,[8,12,13] and (4) ability of nursing staff to implement innovative interventions.[8,10,11,13–16] Three primary interventions were piloted and subsequently implemented house-wide. The first intervention was the use of colored nonskid socks for patients at high risk of falling. The use of yellow socks in addition to a yellow sign posted on door to the patient's room and on the front of the chart alerted other hospital staff that the patient was at high risk of falling. If a patient had fallen in the hospital, he or she received red socks. Anyone seeing a patient in the hall with red socks knew the patient should always be accompanied and not left alone. Second, a safety huddle was added to the change-of-shift communication procedure on each unit. The patients at high risk of falling were identified and labeled as a "community patient." Every staff member was expected to respond immediately to these patients' call lights. Third, for reporting falls, an algorithm was developed that included an immediate fall debriefing. This algorithm provided timely critical information that is often forgotten when reporting is delayed. These interventions created a heightened staff awareness and focus on fall prevention rather than fall-risk assessment. After implementation, the fall rate decreased 18% and the rate of falls with injury was reduced by 30%.

Pressure Ulcer Prevention Best Practice Team

Before the formation of the Pressure Ulcer Best Practice Team, quarterly pressure ulcer prevalence studies showed that rates of hospital-acquired pressure ulcers at St. Luke's were below national benchmarks. Even so, the interdisciplinary team chose to focus on further decreasing this percentage and on addressing prevention. Represented on the team were nursing, pharmacy, physical therapy, and nutrition services. Nursing representatives included staff nurses, nurse managers, advanced practice nurses, and certified wound ostomy nurses. After reviewing the literature, the team found that staff education was the key to a thorough skin assessment and the implementation of interventions to prevent skin breakdown.[17–23] With the assistance of nurse managers from each of the acute and critical care units, staff nurses were identified to be skin resource nurses. These nurses were divided into teams to collect the quarterly pressure ulcer prevalence data. They were given extensive instruction on pressure ulcer staging and interrater reliability was established. In addition, these staff nurses assisted with the further education of staff nurses on the use of the Braden Scale assessment to assess patients at risk of skin breakdown and to implement measures to prevent breakdown based on the Braden subscale assessment.[24] If skin breakdown did occur, staff nurses were instructed about how to describe these pressure ulcers using common terminology, including location, depth, status of wound bed, and appearance of wound edges and surrounding skin. The team also worked with representatives from information systems. Nurses now send reports daily to nutrition indicating which patients have low albumin. Those patients then receive early treatment. An on-line incident report has been developed to facilitate early reporting of skin breakdown. At this writing, the incidence reporting is still being piloted. Pressure ulcer prevalence has decreased since this initiative began. Ulcers equal to or greater than stage II have decreased 18%.

Hand-Off Communication Best Practice Team

The Hand-Off Communication Best Practice Team was established to develop a comprehensive plan for more effective communication hospital-wide. Patients interact with multiple caregivers and departments on a daily basis. During many of these interactions, caregivers make observations or collect data that must be consistently and accurately passed on to other caregivers. To improve the process of sharing information, a team was formed with staff and managers from nursing, perioperative services, diagnostic testing areas, emergency department, transportation, social services, and case management. Hand-off communication is defined as the interactive process of passing patient-specific information from one caregiver to another or from one team of caregivers to another for the purpose of ensuring the continuity and safety of the patient's care.[25] Two related initiatives had already been implemented successfully in nursing. One was the use of the communication technique represented by the acronym SBAR for *situation, background, assessment,* and *recommendation.*[26,27] The technique is designed to ensure that nurses, in communicating with physicians, provide useful and clear information in an efficient way. The nurse first describes the situation, then summarizes the background, then provides an assessment, and finally makes a recommendation. The team recommended that the SBAR technique used successfully by nurses be implemented by caregivers hospital-wide. The other initiative was the use of a universal transfer report upon transfer to another level of care. To exceed the standard outlined in The Joint Commission National Patient Safety Goal #2,[28] the team identified a need for a standardized house-wide approach to hand-off communication that included the opportunity to ask and respond to questions. After an extensive literature review of published best practices on hand-off and team communication, the team created three report forms. The forms are based on the patient's destination and the level of information required. The most comprehensive form is the preoperative checklist,[29] which is the written report and checklist to be completed before the patient entered the operating room. The preprocedure checklist was created for invasive testing and includes an area for a return report to be completed by the staff in the testing department. The third form was the trip ticket that provides a written report for transfer of the patient to a noninvasive testing or examination area. Change-of-shift reporting[30–33] and a verification process before invasive procedures—known as a "time-out"[34,35]—are also critical communication events. A template was created for change-of-shift report. The elements of a "time-out" were identified on a sticker that could be placed in the patient's chart for procedures performed at the bedside. To educate staff, the team produced a video that demonstrated both the use of the change-of-shift report template and how to conduct a proper time-out. The checklists, trip ticket, change-of-shift report, and time-out stickers have improved communication among caregivers and enhanced patient safety. After the initial implementation of the new forms and processes, chart reviews and observations revealed a 89% compliance with the changes. Through ongoing record review and unit rounding, the current compliance is 93%.

SUMMARY

The replacement of the traditional nursing quality council with the Best Practice Council has helped St. Luke's Episcopal Hospital regain the focus of its nursing quality efforts. The structure provided to the teams by the Evidence Based Practice Model gave the hospital a consistent roadmap for solving quality problems. The success of the teams can be attributed to clear directions, an aggressive timeline, and the short-term commitment required of team members. The teams have remained focused and on track. Each team met their original goals. In the spirit of continuous quality improvement—and despite the original plan for them to disband after meeting goals—each team continues to meet and has identified new projects and goals to work toward. Meanwhile, new teams have formed to address additional areas for improvement identified through review of outcomes data by the Best Practice Council.

REFERENCES

1. Titler MG, Klieber C, Steelman V, et al. Infusing research into practice to promote quality care. Nurs Res 1994;43(5):307–13.

2. Melnyk B, Fineout-Overholt E. Evidence based practice in nursing & healthcare: a guide to best practice. Philadelphia (PA): Lippincott, Williams, Wilkins; 2005.

3. National Center for Preparedness D, and Control of Infectious Diseases. National Nosocomial Infections Surveillance System (NNIS). Centers for Disease Control and Prevention. Available at: http://www.cdc.gov/ncidod/dhqp/nnis.html. Accessed June 25, 2008.

4. Improvement IfH. Getting started kit: prevent central line infections. IHI. Available at: http://www.ihi.org/nr/rdonlyres/2ab66d90-c8e0-4a22-82a4-55ea9d93f94e/0/centrallineinfectionsbibliography.doc. Accessed June 25, 2008.

5. O'Grady N, Alexander M, Dellinger E, et al. Guidelines for the prevention of intravascular catheter-related infections. MMWR 2002;51(No. RR-10). Centers for Disease Control and Prevention. Available at: http://www.cdc.gov/mmwr/preview/mmwrhtml/rr5110a1.htm. Accessed June 25, 2008.

6. Wall R, Ely E, Elasy T, et al. Using real time process measurements to reduce catheter related bloodstream infections in the intensive care unit. Qual Saf Health Care 2005;14(4):295–302.

7. Hendrich A. The AHI Fall Prevention Program with the Hendrich II Fall Risk Model©. Available at: http://www.ahincorp.com/hfrm/index.php. Accessed June 25, 2008.

8. Szumlas S, Groszek J, Kitt S, et al. Take a second glance: a novel approach to inpatient fall prevention. Jt Comm J Qual Saf 2004;30(6):295–302.

9. Krauss M, Evanoff B, Hitcho E, et al. A case-control study of patient, medication and care-related risk factors for inpatient falls. J Gen Intern Med 2004;20(2):116–22.

10. Mills P, Neily J, Luan D, et al. Using aggregate root cause analysis to reduce falls and related injuries. Jt Comm J Qual Patient Saf 2005;31(1):21–31.

11. Vassallo M, Vignaraja R, Sharma J, et al. Predictors for falls among hospital inpatients with impaired mobility. J R Soc Med 2004;97(6):266–9.

12. Ray W, Taylor J, Brown A, et al. Prevention of fall-related injuries in long-term care: a randomized controlled trial of staff education. Arch Intern Med 2005;165(19):2293–8.

13. Haines T, Bennell K, Osborne R, et al. Effectiveness of targeted falls prevention programme in subacute hospital setting: randomised controlled trial. BMJ 2004;328(7441):676–82.

14. Jeske L, Kolmer V, Muth M, et al. Partnering with patients and families in designing visual cues to prevent falls in hospitalized elders. J Nurs Care Qual 2006;21(3):236–41.

15. Dempsey J. Falls prevention revisited: a call for a new approach. J Clin Nurs 2004;13(4):479–85.

16. Healey F, Monro A, Cockram A, et al. Using targeted risk factor reduction to prevent falls in older in-patients: a randomised controlled trial. Age Ageing 2004;33(4):390–5.

17. Bryant R, Nix DE. Acute & chronic wounds: current management concepts. 3rd edition. St. Louis (MO): Mosby Elsevier; 2007.

18. Courtney B, Ruppman J, Cooper H. Save our skin: initiative cuts pressure ulcer incidence in half. Nurs Manage 2006;37(4):36–45.

19. Lyder C, Grady J, Mathur D, et al. Preventing pressure ulcers in Connecticut hospitals by using the plan-do-study-act model of quality improvement. Jt Comm J Qual Saf 2004;30(4):205–13.

20. National Pressure Ulcer Advisory Panel. Updated staging system. Available at: http://www.npuap.org/pr2.htm. Accessed October 9, 2007.

21. Scanlon E, Stubbs N. Pressure relieving devices for treating heel pressure ulcers (Protocol). Cochrane Database Syst Rev 2005, 2006;(4):CD005485.10.1002/14651858.

22. Whittington K, Briones R. National prevalence and incidence study: 6-year sequential acute care data. Adv Skin Wound Care 2004;17(9):490–4.
23. Young T, Clark M. Re-positioning for pressure ulcer prevention. (Protocol). Cochrane Database Syst Rev 2003, 2006;(4):CD004836. 10.1002/14651858.
24. Braden B, Bergstrom N. Braden scale for predicting pressure sore risk. Available at: http://www.bradenscale.com/braden.PDF. Accessed June 25, 2008.
25. Joint Commission Resources. Improving handoff communications: Meeting National Patient Safety Goal 2E. Joint Commission International Center for Patient Safety. Accessed June 25, 2008.
26. Kaiser Permanente of Colorado. SBAR technique for communication: a situational briefing model. Institute for Healthcare Improvement. Available at: http://www.ihi. org/IHI/Topics/PatientSafety/SafetyGeneral/Tools/SBARTechniqueforCommunication ASituationalBriefingModel.htm. Accessed June 25, 2008.
27. Haig K, Sutton S, Whittington J. SBAR: a shared mental model for improving communication between clinicians. Jt Comm J Qual Patient Saf 2006;32(3):167–75.
28. National Patient Safety Goals. The Joint Commission. Available at: http://www.jointcommission.org/PatientSafety/NationalPatientSafetyGoals/. Accessed June 25, 2008.
29. Lingard L, Espin S, Rubin B, et al. Getting teams to talk: development and pilot implementation of a checklist to promote interprofessional communication in the OR. Qual Saf Health Care 2005;14(5):340–6.
30. Benson E, Rippin-Sisler C, Jabusch K, et al. Improving nursing shift-to-shift report. J Nurs Care Qual 2007;22(1):80–4.
31. Lamond D. The information content of the nurse change of shift report: a comparative study. J Adv Nurs 2000;31(4):794–804.
32. Strople B, Ottani P. Can technology improve intershift report? What the research reveals. J Prof Nurs 2006;22(3):197–204.
33. Thompson D, Holzmueller C, Hunt D, et al. A morning briefing: setting the stage for a clinically and operationally good day. Jt Comm J Qual Patient Saf 2005; 31(8):476–9.
34. Anonymous. Best practices for preventing wrong site, wrong person, and wrong procedure errors in perioperative settings. AORN J 2006;84(Suppl 1):S13–29.
35. Saufl N. Universal protocol for preventing wrong site, wrong procedure, wrong person surgery. J Perianesth Nurs 2004;19(5):348–51.

Development and Implementation of an Inductive Model for Evidence-Based Practice: A Grassroots Approach for Building Evidence-Based Practice Capacity in Staff Nurses

Tania D. Strout, RN, BSN, MS[a],*, Kelly Lancaster, RN, BSN, CAPA[b],
Alyce A. Schultz, RN, PhD, FAAN[c]

KEYWORDS

- Evidence-based practice • Nursing • Nursing practice
- Clinical scholarship • Clinical scholar • Clinical scholar model

WHAT IS EVIDENCE-BASED PRACTICE?

Sackett and colleagues'[1] definition states that evidence-based practice (EBP) is "the integration of best research evidence with clinical expertise and patient values." Their definition is an important departure from a previous one, "the conscientious, explicit, and judicious use of current best evidence in making decisions about the care of individual patients." The updated approach presents a synergy among three essential components: a research evidence, the expertise of clinicians, and the values of the patients they serve.[2] It acknowledges the tensions that exist in developing a balance

[a] Maine Medical Center, Department of Emergency Medicine, 321 Brackett Street, Portland, ME 04102, USA
[b] Maine Medical Center, Scarborough Surgery Center, 84 Campus Drive, Scarborough, ME 04074, USA
[c] EBP Concepts, Alyce A. Schultz & Associates, LLC, 5747 W. Drake Court, Chandler, AZ 85226, USA
* Corresponding author.
E-mail address: strout@mmc.org (T.D. Strout).

Nurs Clin N Am 44 (2009) 93–102
doi:10.1016/j.cnur.2008.10.007
0029-6465/08/$ – see front matter © 2009 Elsevier Inc. All rights reserved.

between clinical expertise, developed over years of practice at the bedside, and scientific evidence that may or may not be generalizable to patients. This approach also gives credence to a voice formerly silent—that of patients and their families. It takes into account their cultures, ethnicities, ideas about health and wellness, and all the other unique attributes that make them who they are. An additional EBP definition includes concern for feasibility, risk or harm, and costs.[3]

This article discusses the development and implementation of one model for EBP education, the Clinical Scholar Model, within a framework relevant for the practicing clinical nurse.[4]

CULTURAL READINESS

Maine Medical Center (MMC) is a 606-bed tertiary-care referral center hospital located in Portland, Maine currently employing approximately 1500 registered nurses. MMC nurses participate in a shared governance model that encourages participation in nursing councils where information is exchanged and consensus-based decisions are made by clinical and administrative nurses. As noted by Broom and Tilbury,[5] when staff nurses are involved in decision-making processes, they become empowered, engaged, and have a sense of control over their professional practice.

When the Clinical Scholar Model was being developed, many individual nursing research and EBP projects were in process, with small groups of nurse clinicians being mentored through the projects one-on-one by the hospital's nurse researcher. Accolades and recognition for completed projects were mounting, and administrative support for nursing research was growing throughout the institution. In addition, nurses were encouraged to continue this work by interdisciplinary colleagues, who also began to collaborate on many projects.

As described by Kingdon,[6] windows of opportunity for large-scale change can exist when forces align. For MMC, consensus around various clinical problems and consensus around research and EBP as solutions for those problems came together. The developing professional practice environment and the chief nursing officer's commitment to developing the infrastructure necessary to support EBP came together as elements essential for success.[7,8] The alignment of these forces and the emerging Clinical Scholar Model created the cultural readiness necessary to support the catalyzing changes that full implementation of the model would bring.

DEVELOPMENT OF CLINICAL SCHOLAR MODEL

As the environment at Maine Medical Center became increasingly ready for transformational change, it became clear that a larger number of nurses with basic EBP skills would be necessary to act as front-line change agents and mentors within the clinical setting. Many nurses were coming forward with clinical questions deserving consideration; few, however, were prepared to begin to answer these important questions.

Years earlier, the words of Dr. Janelle Krueger planted the seeds for the development of the model. At one of the nation's first nursing research conferences, Dr. Krueger introduced the idea of research as a staff nurse function and promoted the notion that clinical staff are truly in a position to be able to link research and practice.[9] Vital to the formal development of the Clinical Scholar Model were some of the ideas presented in the Conduct and Utilization of Research in Nursing (CURN) project, change theory concepts discussed by Everett Rogers, and the synthesis of ideas about scholarship disseminated by Sigma Theta Tau, International in the *Clinical Scholarship Resource Paper*.[10–12] The wellspring of innovative ideas developed by clinical nurses within the institution, the visionary and creative leadership of the nurse researcher, and administrative support intersected to encourage development of the model.

Early work on the model addressed not only what its goals and essential components would look like but also how the model would be applied in clinical settings. Key competency areas, including literature search, review and critique, research ethics, project design, proposal development, and computer proficiency, were identified. These skills were to be developed in the Clinical Scholar Program, constructed as didactic sessions followed by hands-on time for mentored work and practice by the participants. The initial series of workshops featured lectures delivered by the nurse researcher, other nationally known nurse scholars, and clinical scholars from within the institution.

Essential to the development of the model and workshop series was a strong desire to adhere to the ethical principles of the conduct of research. The interconnectedness of research conduct, quality, and EBP was identified. Ethical obligations to the potential subjects were primary considerations (**Fig. 1**).[3] For example, for each clinical

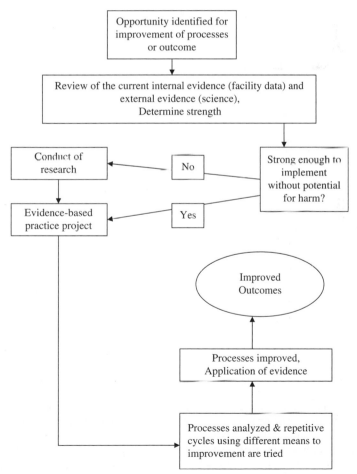

Fig. 1. Interrelationship between research, EBP, and quality. (*Courtesy of* Alyce A. Schultz RN, PhD, FAAN, Chandler, AZ.)

question or potential project, a comprehensive review of the current scientific literature was conducted. When strong and pertinent evidence for a particular practice was present in the literature, nurses were encouraged not to conduct additional research activities but to undertake projects aimed at applying existing evidence to practice and evaluating outcomes following the change. The program's developers and participants believe that it is their ethical obligation to minimize risk to potential subjects by conducting research only when it is truly necessary and to honor the contributions of previous research subjects by applying evidence gained through their participation where appropriate. Nurses participating in the Clinical Scholar Program were strongly encouraged to seek institutional review board review for all nursing EBP and quality improvement projects to ensure compliance and to retain the ability to share results outside of their own institution.

THE MODEL
Description of the Clinical Scholar Model

The Clinical Scholar Model is predicated on the development of a cadre of point-of-care nurses who become clinical scholars, committed to patient care, knowledge development, research translation, and evidence implementation. **Fig. 2** depicts the Clinical Scholar Model used by nurse scholars in the conduct of their research, EBP, and quality improvement projects.

Goals of the Clinical Scholar Model

The Clinical Scholar Model incorporates four central goals. The first is to challenge current practices within the discipline of nursing.[9] The second goal is for clinical nurses to be able to speak and understand the language of research, featuring research-related discussion as a component of day-to-day dialogue. Third, the model seeks to encourage the critical appraisal, critique, and synthesis of current evidence. The final goal of the model is for clinical scholars to serve as mentors to other staff nurses involved in journeys to scholarship through the creation of mentoring partnerships between experienced and novice scholars. The structure provided by these goals is important in providing clarity of purpose and a sense of direction for those working within the model's framework.

Essential Components of the Clinical Scholar Model

The essential components of the model are grounded in the Sigma Theta Tau, International *Clinical Scholarship Resource Paper*.[9,12] It requires the use of observation and scientifically based methods to identify and solve clinical problems. Clinical scholars must analyze both internal and external evidence that substantiates or refutes a current practice. Evidence is synthesized by evaluating its level, quality, quantity, consistency, and strength. Findings are applied, and results are disseminated in poster and oral presentations as well as in the published scientific literature.

IMPLEMENTATION OF THE CLINICAL SCHOLAR MODEL

Implementation of the Clinical Scholar Model began with the development of a series of Clinical Scholar workshops. Ten clinical nurses and the nurse researcher worked to organize and implement six full-day workshops aimed at providing other nurses the knowledge to with which they could begin to develop their own scholarship-in-practice. While the clinicians learned basic evidence-based practice skills, the nurse-mentors learned new methods for knowledge sharing and developing the mentor–mentee relationship and continued to develop their own EBP skills.

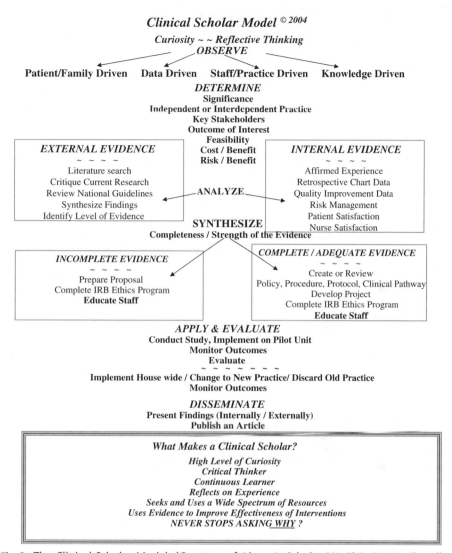

Fig. 2. The Clinical Scholar Model. (*Courtesy of* Alyce A. Schultz RN, PhD, FAAN, Chandler, AZ.)

Because each workshop day was designed to include both didactic and practical time, participants spent a portion of each session applying the skills they had just reviewed. Practical time was conducted within a small-group framework and was facilitated by the nurse mentors. Group discussion, team collaboration, and experiential sharing were encouraged, particularly with review and debriefing at the end of each day. To promote continued practice and project development during the time between workshops, homework assignments were chosen to reinforce and challenge newly developed skills.

At the conclusion of the workshop series, each emerging scholar produced and delivered an oral presentation describing the project he/she had developed during the year. By the end of the first set of workshops, 14 new nursing research, EBP, or quality improvement projects had emerged. These projects ultimately were completed and resulted in many national and international poster and podium presentations, as well as in multiple scientific publications. Several projects received awards from discipline-specific nursing organizations. Most importantly, the results of the different projects were incorporated into daily clinical practice and were adopted by nurses on many units throughout the institution. Along with the integration of these practice changes, EBP and clinical scholarship truly became woven into the tapestry of nursing practice at MMC.

All major change initiatives require administrative support for lasting success, and the Clinical Scholar Model is no exception. Administrators in the department of nursing were invested in and supportive of the development and implementation of this model. Funding for the workshops, including costs for external speaker honoraria, refreshments, and printing, came from the department of nursing and research institute budgets. In addition, funding for workshop attendees was required from the individual nursing units. Each participant was supported with 8 hours of paid time to attend the scheduled workshops and 4 additional hours per month to complete project work. Given that 50 nurses attended the first series of workshops and that replacements needed to be hired to cover nurses' scheduled clinical duties, the contributions of the nursing units were substantial. Clearly, these activities were seen as being in alignment with the institutional values and initiatives.

WHO IS THE CLINICAL SCHOLAR?

Sigma Theta Tau's *Clinical Scholarship Resource Paper* describes clinical scholarship as[12]

> an approach that enables evidence-based nursing and development of best practices to meet the needs of clients efficiently and effectively. It requires the identification of desired outcomes; the use of systematic observation and scientifically based methods to identify and solve clinical problems; the substantiation of practice and clinical decisions with reference to scientific principles, current research, consensus-based guidelines, quality improvement data, and other forms of evidence; the evaluation, documentation, and dissemination of outcomes and improvements in practice through a variety of mechanisms including publication, presentations, consultation, and leadership; and the use of clinical knowledge and expertise to anticipate trends, predict needs, create effective clinical products and services, and manage outcomes.

Clinical scholars connect with these words; they are at the core of their identities as nurses. They are a piece of the scholars' daily functioning: meeting needs effectively, substantiating practice, using evidence, and managing outcomes. As nurses evolve as clinical scholars, the symbiotic relationship between scholarship and practice becomes rich and nourished.

What does the clinical scholar look like? What distinguishes his/her practice? The clinical scholar possesses a high level of curiosity. S/he is the nurse on the unit who not only questions traditional practices and wonders how a practice could be done better next time but deliberates over whether a practice needs to be performed at all. S/he thinks critically to solve complex problems and is not satisfied with a temporary fix. Clinical scholars make time to reflect on their practice, because this activity renews the professional spirit and generates clarity of purpose.

Clinical scholars seek out and use a wide variety of resources in their work, drawing on expert clinicians and scholars alike. They use both internal and external evidence to improve the effectiveness of their interventions, and they find creative ways to incorporate clinical expertise and patient preferences into their care. Most importantly, clinical scholars possess a passion for learning, are never satisfied with the status quo, and never stop asking, "Why?": "Why do we remove intravenous lines based on their time in situ?" "Why don't we use buffered lidocaine for our intravenous starts?" "Why do our open-heart patients recall being intubated?" These are all examples of questions explored by clinical scholars at MMC.

Importantly, as Dr. Melanie Dreher explained in the *Clinical Scholarship Resource Paper*, clinical scholarship is not the same thing as clinical proficiency.[12] She writes that performing a nursing procedure well, even with expertise, does not make it scholarly unless the practitioner also is questioning whether the procedure needs to be performed in the first place or whether there is a better way to accomplish the same objective. Clinical scholarship involves inquiry and a willingness to scrutinize one's own practice. It involves looking for a better way and refusing to accept any practice simply because it has always been done in a particular way.

Clinical scholars are some of nursing's most transformational leaders. They have a vision for the future of health care that excites and converts followers; they can see the big picture and work to help others share in this vision. They sell and model their vision of improved outcomes in their daily actions, both on and off their units. They are invested in this goal and work to bring their patient's agendas forward, but they also recognize and accept the inevitable challenges and setbacks that happen along the way. Clinical scholars face these obstacles with poise and grace. They create trust. They are expert at forging new relationships. They are charismatic, confident, and believe fully in themselves. Clinical scholars are constantly at the forefront; they are innovators who create the path and always can be depended upon to lead the charge. Their commitment to all that they do is unwavering, and they remember take time to provide others with praise, support, and rewards. Clinical scholars live the words of Mahatma Gandhi, "We must be the change we wish to see in the world."

SUSTAINING THE CLINICAL SCHOLAR MODEL

Through its focus on the development of new clinical scholars who can act as EBP mentors to their colleagues in the future, the Clinical Scholar Model is self sustaining. The Clinical Scholar workshops provide a nurturing, rich environment for nurses to create and develop extended networks of professional contacts and colleagues to draw upon for future mentoring. In return for this gift of professional growth, many scholars embrace the opportunity to "pay it forward" by assisting others in their own journeys while continuing to refine their own skill sets through new projects.

Incorporating basic principles of change theory also can assist in sustaining the Clinical Scholar Model. Everett Rogers'[11] *Diffusion of Innovations* provides a useful framework for considering the spread of evidence adoption through health care organizations. His work suggests that innovative change spreads through a society (in this case a health care organization) in an S-shaped curve, with early adopters incorporating the technology first, early and late majorities adopting the innovation next, followed by the final 16% of the population known as "laggards." He further theorized that the rate or speed of technology adoption is affected by the speed at which the adoption takes off and the speed at which later growth occurs. The intensity of the Clinical Scholar Program and the relatively fast pace at which an initial group of clinicians can be educated supports a speedy initial adoption of EBP. The steadier, consistent pace at which those initial clinical scholars act as mentors to new groups reinforces constant growth in the model and supports its continuation in a given organization.

Change theory gives additional assistance by anticipating and planning for resistance to innovation during individual projects and to the new and expanded roles fulfilled by nurses participating in scholarship programs. Completing a probability of adoption assessment, as outlined by the CURN project, is one way to begin thinking about potential sources of resistance to change. The CURN authors also provide useful insights into organizational change, for creating a climate prepared for change, and identifying sources of resistance to change that can be applied with the Clinical Scholar Model.[10]

Maintaining a focus on improvement in patient- and family-centered outcomes also helps sustain the Clinical Scholar Model. Although projects may revolve around issues of importance to nursing as a discipline (eg, on retaining nurses or on nursing education), most concentrate on improving health-related outcomes for patients. When outcomes remain measurable and focused in a way that is so central to the institutional mission of care provision, administrative leaders and clinicians alike can see the value in and give support to the program.

Demonstrating and celebrating programmatic benefits and the benefits of EBP is another effective means of creating support for and sustaining interest in the Clinical Scholar Model. Sharing specific project results at a nursing research day, spreading the news of abstracts presented or awards received, and highlighting successes of the workshops as a whole focuses positive attention on the program. This attention sustains support for the model by creating buy-in from leadership and by providing positive reinforcement for those who will serve as mentors in the future. In addition, recognizing contributions to important programs such as the Magnet Recognition program and the National Database of Nursing Quality Indicators garners support for and sustains the model.

In today's environment of limited health care budgets, financial support for programs such as the Clinical Scholar Model can be limited. Financial investment in the program is essential, and clinical nurses can work successfully toward funding individual projects in support of the larger model. Consideration of the financial implications of any project is an important step in evaluating the probability of adoption of the practice. Evaluating the monetary costs of projects and interventions is essential, and including financial outcomes data whenever possible is a key to providing evidence of benefit in this area. In seeking project funding, clinical nurses without advanced training and with limited access to nurses who have advanced degrees can form creative partnerships with local universities or schools of nursing; these environments are rich with academically prepared nurses who are willing to mentor in this area.

CLINICAL EXEMPLAR: AN EVIDENCE-BASED PRACTICE PROJECT
Observing

Traditionally, criteria for ambulatory surgical discharge have required that patients take oral fluids before discharge home. Nurses in the ambulatory surgery unit at MMC encouraged early intake of oral fluids to ensure that patients met discharge criteria. This practice often led to postoperative nausea and vomiting and frequent use of expensive rescue antiemetics. Additional sequelae were a requirement for increased nursing care hours and delayed discharge for patients.

Frequently, nursing staff would contact physician colleagues to obtain permission to discharge patients without any significant oral fluid intake, providing that patients met the remaining discharge criteria. With the use of shorter-acting anesthetics, many patients were ready for discharge before they were thirsty or ready to drink. The requirement for taking oral fluids was not clearly defined and resulted in wide variations in practice among physicians and nursing staff. Frustrated with the lack of a standardized practice, nurses frequently found themselves asking why they were continuing a practice that seemed to be a source of dissatisfaction for patients, families, and staff alike.

Analyzing

A team of three nurses from the ambulatory surgery unit participated in the Clinical Scholar Program to learn the skills necessary to initiate a practice change, in this case to define further the practice regarding the necessity of mandatory oral fluid intake following ambulatory surgery. Using the Clinical Scholar Model as a framework for supporting the work, the team searched the external evidence for published studies that determined the relevance of oral intake as discharge criteria for adult and pediatric patients. The search yielded five studies and one published clinical guideline. Team members reviewed and critiqued the national guidelines and determined the strength of the published research using a critique form.[13] The internal evidence consisted of anecdotal reports describing patient, family, and nurse experiences and satisfaction; this qualitative evidence was included as part of the group's analysis.

Synthesizing

The outcome variables reviewed in the selected studies included the occurrence of emesis, length of stay, and postoperative complications. The study findings indicated that without mandatory oral intake, there was reduced postoperative vomiting, reduced length of stay, and no significant difference in complications during the first 24 hours following discharge. The project team determined that there was adequate evidence to move forward and make a policy change in discharge criteria.

The MMC ambulatory surgery discharge criteria were updated to reflect the evidence. Oral fluid intake became optional, with exceptions made by physician prescription. Patients needed to demonstrate the ability to swallow and were evaluated for minimal nausea and vomiting before discharge. Nursing staff no longer forced oral fluid intake against patients' wishes or delayed discharge for lack of oral intake.

Applying and Evaluating

Following the policy update and staff education, the practice change was implemented in the ambulatory surgery unit. Quality improvement data were collected, and outcomes were monitored. Evaluation of data after implementation demonstrated no negative outcomes related to the elimination of mandatory oral fluid intake following ambulatory surgery.

Disseminating

The findings from this project were presented to the ambulatory surgery unit and to the MMC community at an annual Nursing Research Conference and to the larger nursing community at a statewide conference. As a result of experience gained in the Clinical Scholar Program, staff nurses were able to identify a clinical issue and make a change that led to positive outcomes for patients, their families, and their nursing colleagues. This success fueled continued motivation for development as clinical scholars. MMC ambulatory surgery nurses now have the knowledge and expertise to use EBP to improve patient outcomes.

SUMMARY

EBP is an essential component of the development of nursing science and has importance for today's clinical nurses. It benefits patients, organizations, and the nursing discipline, as well as having personal and professional benefits for individual clinicians. As interest in EBP has grown, so has the need for educational programs designed to develop the scholarly skills of the nursing workforce. The Clinical Scholar Model is one grassroots approach to developing a cadre of clinical nurses with the EBP and research skills necessary in today's demanding health care delivery environments.

ACKNOWLEDGMENT

The authors acknowledge the generous support of the department of nursing at Maine Medical Center during the development and implementation of this work. Without the backing of our nursing administrators, managers, and clinician colleagues, this work would not have been possible; to each of them we offer our most sincere thanks. In addition, we offer our thanks to the nurses, patients, and physicians who collaborated on the mandatory oral hydration project.

REFERENCES

1. Sackett DL, Straus SE, Richardson WS, et al, editors. Evidence-based medicine—how to practice and teach EBP. New York: Churchill Livingstone; 2000.
2. Sackett DL, Rosenberg WM, Gray JA, et al. Evidence based medicine: what it is and what it isn't. BMJ 1996;312(7023):71–2.
3. Schultz AA. Research, evidence-based practice, and quality improvement in a clinical setting. Phoenix (AZ): Alyce A. Schultz; 2007.
4. Schultz AA. Clinical scholars at the bedside: an EBP mentorship model for today. ENK: Excellence in Nursing Knowledge Feb 2005.
5. Broom CM, Tilbury MS. Magnet status: a journey not a destination. J Nurs Care Qual 2007;22(2):113–8.
6. Kingdon JW. Bridging research and policy: agendas, alternatives, and public policies. New York: Harper Collins; 1984.
7. Titler MG, Everett LQ. Sustain an infrastructure to support EBP. Nurs Manage 2006; 37(9):14–6.
8. Stetler CB, Brunell M, Giuliano KK, et al. Evidence-based practice and the role of nursing leadership. J Nurs Adm 1998;28(7/8):45–53.
9. Schultz AA. Origins and aspirations: conceiving the clinical scholar model. ENK: Excellence in nursing knowledge 2005.
10. Horsley JA, Crane J, Crabtree MK, et al. Using research to improve nursing practice: a guide. Philadelphia: WB Saunders Company; 1983.
11. Rogers EM. Diffusion of innovations. 5th edition. New York: Free Press; 2003.
12. Clinical Scholarship Task Force, Sigma Theta Tau International. Clinical scholar resource paper 1999. Available at: wwwnursingsociety.org. Accessed April 9, 2008.
13. Gallant P. Analysis: what's all the speak about critique? ENK: Excellence in Nursing Knowledge 2005.

Effect of a Preoperative Instructional Digital Video Disc on Patient Knowledge and Preparedness for Engaging in Postoperative Care Activities

Joe Ong, RN, BSN[a], Pamela S. Miller, RN, PhD(c), ACNP, CNS[b],
Renee Appleby, RN[a], Rebecca Allegretto, RN, BSN[c],
Anna Gawlinski, RN, DNSc, CS-ACNP[a,]*

KEYWORDS

- Patient education • Preoperative instructional digital video disc
- Evidence-based practice

Health care delivery systems have been restructured in recent years to focus on achieving high-quality outcomes for patients by using the most cost-effective methods.[1] Optimizing outcomes for patients undergoing surgery requires the collaborative and coordinated efforts of physicians, nurses, and allied health personnel.[2] Preoperative teaching serves as a standard of nursing practice within the surgical setting.[3] Providing patients with supportive preoperative teaching that incorporates the most useful information about postoperative activities within a confined time frame has been a challenge.[1] The psychologic burden placed on patients in the preoperative

This work was supported by funding provided by the Ronald Reagan University of California Los Angeles Women's Auxillary.

[a] Department of Nursing, Ronald Reagan University of California Los Angeles Medical Center, Los Angeles, CA 90095, USA

[b] University of Los Angeles School of Nursing, Los Angeles, CA 90095, USA

[c] Thoracic Surgery, Ronald Reagan University of California Los Angeles Medical Center, Los Angeles, CA 90095, USA

* Corresponding author. Ronald Reagan University of California Los Angeles Medical Center, Los Angeles, CA 90095, USA.

E-mail address: agawlinski@mednet.ucla.edu (A. Gawlinski).

period may be underestimated, and this burden lessens patients' ability to comprehend and contribute to the postsurgical plan. Patients have a defined learning curve for understanding the intricacies of the surgical procedure and facilitating their own recovery after surgery. The effectiveness of preoperative teaching depends, in part, on the learning needs, style, and preference of the patient. The amount of information conferred to patients may be overwhelming.[2] As a result, the patient may require repeated or frequent reinforcement. Once the patient has had the opportunity to grasp the information, additional questions may arise. Nurses are in a key position to provide preoperative teaching and respond to patients' questions and concerns.[2] Advancements in technology have provided nurses with the opportunity to improve and intensify preoperative educational strategies.

SCOPE OF THE PROBLEM IN EXISTING PRACTICE

In general, preoperative teaching should include significant information about the surgery and issues that patients are anticipated to face in the perioperative and postoperative periods. Surgical procedures expose patients to pain, bodily injury, and potential death.[4] Preoperative teaching readily and effectively enables patients to cope with their surgery, reduces the duration of hospitalization, elevates satisfaction, minimizes postsurgical complications, and augments patients' psychologic well-being.[4]

Preoperative teaching has been administered in various ways and formats:[2] verbal instruction, printed materials, demonstrations, and videotapes. Routine dissemination of information by means of verbal instruction with supplemental written material (information packets) has been the basis for preoperative teaching for decades. Such factors as degree of attentiveness, emotional aptitude, intellectual level, learning disabilities, and language or cultural barriers can affect patients' ability to assimilate the information.[2]

Currently, substantive inconsistencies are apparent in preoperative instruction for thoracic surgical patients who are scheduled to undergo such procedures as esophagectomy or lung volume reduction surgery. Ideally, a written preoperative instructional handout was to be given during each patient's preoperative surgical visit. Baseline data indicated that 23 (92%) of 25 patients did not receive the written handout. This lapse has resulted in a lack of knowledge and preparedness that prevents patients from immediately engaging successfully in postoperative self-care activities (eg, ambulation and pain management), which can lead to increases in patients' anxiety, postoperative complications, and length of stay in the hospital. Thus, the challenge was to develop structures and processes that would enable thoracic surgical patients to receive thorough preoperative teaching consistently.

An evidence-based project that included development of postoperative thoracic surgery information in a standardized format by using state-of-the-art digital video disc (DVD) technology was implemented. This staff nurse–driven project illustrates the contribution of preoperative teaching to improving patients' outcomes. The evidence-based literature and the evaluation of an audiovisual medium dedicated to providing patients with valuable information on the spectrum of care activities after thoracic surgery are discussed.

EVIDENCE-BASED LITERATURE

Preoperative teaching has been defined in the literature as an "interactive process of providing information and explanations about surgical processes, expected patient behaviors, and anticipated sensations and providing appropriate reassurance...to patients who are about to undergo surgery."[1] Postoperative care refers to nursing activities performed during the patient's postoperative phase. Preoperative teaching not only provides patient-specific information about what to expect during the postoperative period but influences the attitudes and behaviors of patients with respect to their postoperative care.[1,5]

Little experimental or quasiexperimental research has explored the impact of preoperative instruction in patients undergoing thoracic surgery. Most studies have explored its impact among selected patients undergoing such procedures as cardiac surgery,[6] orthopedic surgery,[7] reproductive surgery,[4] and cancer surgery.[8] Published reports describe a positive relation between preoperative teaching and improved outcomes for patients and indicate that preoperative teaching is a cost-effective approach.[7] **Table 1** lists the relevant studies reviewed for this project and their respective level of evidence.

In a qualitative study by Doering and colleagues[6] of patients' perceptions of the quality of nursing and medical care during hospitalization after cardiac surgery, patients wanted to know what they could honestly and realistically expect during their postoperative recovery. Specific information embedded within the preoperative education provided by nurses can assist patients in understanding the level of their participation that is required during recovery. Meeting the informational and physical needs of patients is imperative.[6] Well-informed patients are more likely to experience positive outcomes and to have higher levels of satisfaction with their care. Such patients have the confidence to carry out behaviors necessary for successful postoperative outcomes.[4] Additional evidence supports the use of video-teaching versus routine care: video-teaching resulted in decreases in postoperative complications (eg, atelectasis) and length of stay among patients undergoing coronary artery bypass graft surgery.[9]

Stern and Lockwood[10] conducted a systematic review of randomized controlled trials investigating preoperative instruction of patients and the effect of such instruction on patients' understanding of, knowledge of, and ability to perform postoperative activities. On the basis of limited rigorous studies, these researchers concluded that preoperative teaching before admission and the use of preoperative videos improved patients' knowledge and skill.[10]

The teaching must take into consideration the emotional state of the patient and the patient's ability to cope,[11] factors that often may be overshadowed by feelings of anxiety or fear about the impending procedure.[2] The evidence supports the benefit of preoperative teaching in reducing anxiety and complications and in improving recovery. Studies have shown an inverse relation between preoperative teaching and postoperative anxiety, wherein improved outcomes were exemplified not only by lower levels of anxiety but by shorter stays in the hospital.[12]

Brumfield and colleagues[5] conducted a descriptive study to isolate important content areas in preoperative teaching as reported by patients and nurses in ambulatory surgery settings. Patients and nurses strongly favored the inclusion of situational information (eg, explaining activities, explaining events), patient role information (eg, anticipated behaviors), and psychosocial support (eg, emotional descriptors) in preoperative teaching. Patients undergoing ambulatory surgery preferred for this teaching to occur before admission. Early instruction targeted toward patients' priorities seems to be critical to enhancing postoperative outcomes.[5] Similar needs of patients were identified in the inpatient surgical setting.[13]

Fitzpatrick and Hyde[14] reported that nurse-related factors, such as individual knowledge and experience, may influence the preoperative education received by patients. This influence is particularly evident among novice nurses or nurses who are new to the clinic or unit. The diversity in degree of knowledge and experience

Table 1
Levels of evidence for the review of the literature

Authors	Level of Evidence
Bernier and colleagues, 2003	Level V: evidence from observational studies with consistent results (eg, correlational, descriptive studies)
Whyte and Grant, 2005	Level VI: evidence from expert opinion, multiple case reports, or national consensus reports
Lewis and colleagues, 2002	Level V: evidence from observational studies with consistent results (eg, correlational, descriptive studies)
Oetker-Black and colleagues, 2003	Level II: evidence from one or more randomized controlled trials with consistent results
Brumfield, and colleagues, 1996	Level V: evidence from observational studies with consistent results (eg, correlational, descriptive studies)
Doering and colleagues, 2002	Level V: evidence from observational studies with consistent results (eg, correlational, descriptive studies)
Johansson and colleagues, 2005	Level I: evidence from well-designed data meta-analysis or well-done systematic review with results that consistently support a specific action (eg, assessment, intervention, or treatment)
Evrard and colleagues, 2005	Level V: evidence from observational studies with consistent results (eg, correlational, descriptive studies)
Shaban and colleagues, 2002	Level IV: evidence from one or more quasiexperimental studies with consistent results
Stern and Lockwood, 2005	Level I: evidence from well-designed data meta-analysis or well-done systematic review with results that consistently support a specific action (eg, assessment, intervention, or treatment)
Doering and colleagues, 2000	Level II: evidence from one or more randomized controlled trials with consistent results
Devine and Cook, 1983	Level I: evidence from well-designed data meta-analysis or well-done systematic review with results that consistently support a specific action (eg, assessment, intervention, or treatment)
Yount and Schoessler, 1991	Level V: evidence from observational studies with consistent results (eg, correlational, descriptive studies)
Fitzpatrick and Hyde, 2006	Level V: evidence from observational studies with consistent results (eg, correlational, descriptive studies)
Thomas and colleagues, 1999	Level V: evidence from observational studies with consistent results (eg, correlational, descriptive studies)
Hathaway, 1986	Level I: evidence from well-designed data meta-analysis or well-done systematic review with results that consistently support a specific action (eg, assessment, intervention, or treatment)

possessed by nurses can produce inconsistent and ineffective preoperative preparation for patients. Addressing this challenge requires an organizational commitment to address internal practices[14] and might best be accomplished through structured preoperative education across the board.

Evrard and colleagues[8] surveyed 108 postsurgical oncology patients who had watched a preoperative DVD. The DVD content included general information pertaining to the hospital environment and postoperative complications in addition to specialized surgery-specific information. The survey asked patients to evaluate the following DVD content areas: (1) access to the information, (2) presentation, (3) patients' perception, and (4) global satisfaction. Seventy-one percent of the patients reported that the DVD provided a positive and encouraging experience, and 83% recommended its use as a preoperative teaching tool. Interestingly, among the 14 patients who experienced complications, only 21% thought that they had received thorough information from the DVD and only 12% believed that they were well prepared to handle postoperative complications. Notably, the patients were allowed to view the DVD only in the clinical setting and were unable to take the DVD home to review. This limitation undermines any chance for patients to reinforce the information and improve recall.[8]

Earlier research using meta-analyses (eg, Hathaway[15]) supported the value of traditional preoperative instruction to improve postoperative outcomes. Modern-day video technology has emerged as a suitable tool for relaying practical information in a timely manner. The visual and auditory emphasis of standardized educational videos provides an additive effect to traditional written preoperative instruction, an additive effect that increases recall.[16] Use of audiovisual materials, such as DVDs, benefits patients because they are able to refer back to and review the information at their convenience. The richness of this multimedia tool provides a venue for answering basic questions that come up after preoperative discussions with the surgeon or nurses. The timing of teaching is best when the DVD is viewed at home before the surgical procedure, in a less stressful environment. Preoperative teaching should be provided near the time of surgery. Teaching should not be provided too early; otherwise, patients are more likely to forget.

PURPOSE OF EVIDENCE-BASED PROJECT

The purpose of this evidence-based practice project was to determine the effects of developing and implementing an innovative preoperative instructional DVD on patients' level of knowledge, preparedness, and perceived ability to participate in postoperative care activities at a university-affiliated public medical center.

INTERVENTION FOR PROJECT IMPLEMENTATION

After gaps in existing preoperative teaching practice were identified and the literature was reviewed, this project was developed on the basis of the principles identified in the Iowa Model of Evidence-Based Practice.[17] The design used convenience sampling methods to survey a group of registered nurses from the medical observation unit before and after the intervention and to survey a group of thoracic surgical patients after the intervention.

This project had two intervention phases. The first intervention was to redesign the delivery of preoperative instruction by developing a preoperative instructional DVD for thoracic surgical patients that was evidence-based and prepared patients to engage in postoperative care activities. The staff nurse collaborated with the director of the medical observation unit on developing the DVD. Thoracic surgeons, clinic staff, and the nurse specialist were consulted about the content of the video. The development of the DVD necessitated scripting, filming, editing, and replication. Partnership with a production crew resulted in the production of a user-friendly DVD. The following content areas of the preoperative teaching program were incorporated into the instructional DVD: pain management, surgical drainage, vital signs, incentive spirometry (IS), cough and deep breathing, chest physiotherapy (CPT), TED hose (antiembolism stockings)/sequential compression device (SCD), ambulation, diet/bowel activity/urine output, and discharge. Patients and staff nurses from the medical observation unit and thoracic surgeons were participants in the DVD. The final DVD was reviewed and approved by all key persons who had a stake in the process.

The second phase of the intervention implemented the delivery process for the preoperative instructional DVD to be given to patients. The system was changed to ensure that all patients were consistently provided with a preoperative instructional DVD. The staff nurse worked in partnership with the clinic staff and nurse specialist to assist in providing patients with the DVD and obtaining survey results. All nursing personnel involved in preoperative teaching and postoperative patient care were taught about the project and inclusion of the DVD. This process included providing each thoracic surgical patient with a preoperative packet during the preoperative clinic visit. The packet included a copy of the 14-minute DVD and a written survey to evaluate the patient's self-reported knowledge and preparedness for surgery. Patients were provided mailing instructions to return the completed survey. Nurses were instructed to complete surveys before and after the intervention that documented the nurses' assessment of patients' knowledge and preparedness to engage in postoperative care activities.

POSTINTERVENTION RESULTS

Data were analyzed by using descriptive statistics and Student's t tests.

Registered Nurses

Before and after the intervention, registered nurses completed a six-item survey to assess patients' knowledge of and preparedness to engage in postoperative care activities. The survey included questions related to the nurses' demographic characteristics.

Demographic characteristics of the 18 registered nurse participants indicated that most of the nurses were female (n = 16 [89%]) and rotated between the day shift and night shift (n = 16 [89%]). Most nurses possessed between 1 and 5 years of total nursing experience (n = 16 [89%]) and had between 1 and 5 years of experience in the medical observation unit of the University of California, Los Angeles (UCLA; n = 15 [83%]). At the time of the project, nearly all nurses served as a clinical nurse level II on the clinical ladder system (Table 2).

Based on the Likert scale (1 = not knowledgeable to 4 = very knowledgeable), nurses' response to the question "How knowledgeable do you feel your thoracic surgical patients were about each of the following important aspects of postoperative care?" indicated a significantly higher level of knowledge after the intervention for aspects of surgical drainage, IS, cough and deep breathing, and TED hose/SCDs (z = −3.461, −2.899, −3.095, and −2.960, respectively; $P \leq .004$; Fig. 1). Nurses also reported significant increases in knowledge about general care (mean: 1.94 versus 3.06; $P < .001$) and pain management (mean: 2.17 versus 3.22; $P < .001$) after the intervention.

Based on the Likert scale (1 = not engaged to 4 = very engaged), nurses' response to the question "How engaged do you feel your thoracic surgical patients were about

Table 2
Demographic characteristics of the nurses who completed surveys before and after the intervention

Variable	Sample (N = 18)	%
Title		
Clinical nurse I	1	5.6
Clinical nurse II	16	88.9
Clinical nurse III	1	5.6
Shift		
Days	1	5.6
Nights	1	5.6
Rotate	16	88.9
Gender		
Male	2	11.1
Female	16	88.9
Years of nursing experience		
<1	1	5.6
1–5	16	88.9
>10	1	5.6
Years of experience in the UCLA medical observation unit		
<1	2	11.1
1–5	15	83.3
6–10	1	5.6

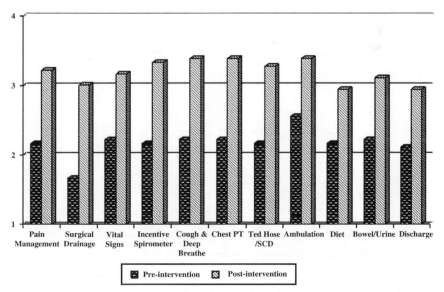

Fig. 1. Mean level of patients' knowledge of postoperative care activities reported by nurses surveyed before and after the intervention. Asterisks indicate significant difference ($P<.004$) from before to after the intervention. PT, physiotherapy.

each of the following important aspects of postoperative care?" indicated a significantly higher level of understanding after the intervention for aspects of IS, cough and deep breathing, and TED hose/SCDs ($z = -3.411, -3.255$, and -2.804, respectively; $P \leq .007$; **Fig. 2**). Nurses reported a significant increase in overall knowledge of patients and engagement of patients and their families ($P \leq .004$).

Nurses were provided with the opportunity to respond with comments at the end of the survey. **Box 1** and **2** cite a few of the nurses' anecdotal comments before the intervention and after the intervention respectively. Responses are best summed up by the response of one nurse who stated that "Giving patients/family members information regarding what to expect of them in regards to postoperation activities will empower them to be in control of their care."

Patients Undergoing Thoracic Surgery

After a review of the DVD, patients were surveyed for their knowledge and perceived ability to participate in postoperative care activities. Patients (n = 15) who participated in this project were predominantly older than 60 years of age (n = 12 [80%]) and English-speaking (n = 14 [93%]). Fifty-three percent were female (n = 8), and 47% were male (n = 7). Most patients had undergone lung surgery (**Table 3**).

Based on the Likert scale (1 = I do not understand to 4 = I understand very well), on the postintervention survey, patients' response to the question "How much do you understand about each of the following after viewing the preoperative DVD?" indicated

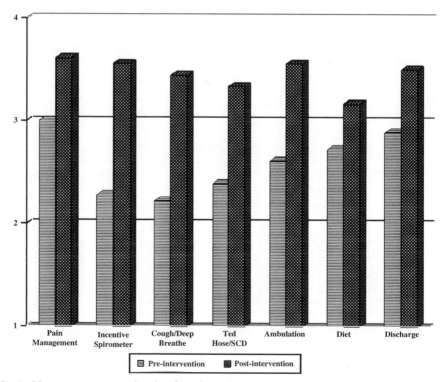

Fig. 2. Mean engagement levels of patients in postoperative care activities reported by nurses surveyed before and after the intervention. Asterisks indicate significant difference (*P*<.007) from before to after the intervention.

Table 3
Demographic characteristics of the patients undergoing thoracic surgery who completed surveys after the intervention

Variable	No. (N = 15)	%
Age, years		
18–30	1	6.7
31–40	1	6.7
41–60	1	6.7
>60	12	80.0
Gender		
Male	7	46.7
Female	8	53.3
Primary language		
English	14	93.3
Other	1	6.7
Type of surgery		
Esophageal	1	6.7
Lung	10	66.7
Other	3	20.0

Box 1
Comments by nurses before the intervention

- "We need to properly evaluate whether the thoracic patient and family have fully understood the concepts and components of postoperative care. It's not enough for the person giving the instructions to hand out pamphlets as reading materials to patients and assume that they'll follow them postoperatively."

- "Patients usually do not expect to walk three times daily and are surprised as to how much work we want them to do. Teaching them preoperatively about the post-op activities would be beneficial. The whiteboards marking their progress with ambulation, CPT, and IS (like a scoreboard) also help to remind them of these activities. Letting them know that the family can help also assists in getting activity done. Most times, the family is unsure of where they can help. Specifically telling them they can assist with CPT and IS engages them more in patient care. Visual demos—most helpful in telling patients, for example, to inflate lungs with the IS."

- "Patients...post-op 3 or 2...still do not know much of any of their post-op therapies or if they did not know, they did not know why they were doing what they were doing. They were sort of knowledgeable of the purposes of the SCDs and TEDs, but the incentive spirometer, they would just breathe in real fast and they said they were exercising their lungs but when demonstrating how to do it, they were just breathing in and out really fast. When I did chest PT, I asked if they know why I was doing it and they all said they did not know. But after instruction that it is to loosen up secretions, they were more enthusiastic to do it."

- "Educated in the medicating...This is not to intimidate the patient/family but to empower them from the very beginning."

- "Patients and their families need reinforcement when it comes to teaching. Although they are somewhat knowledgeable overall, they need to be reminded to follow through with post-op care."

> **Box 2**
> **Comments by nurses after the intervention**
>
> - "The instructional DVD was very useful in educating thoracic patients with regards to their role and expectations after surgery."
> - "Patients as well as family were very knowledgeable about pain medication, CPT, IS, Ambulation . . . . Relatives were very involved in patients' care."
> - "This DVD was very helpful in preparing patients in becoming familiar with what to expect after surgery. When the nurses did their teaching it was nice when the patient and/or family members were not hearing things for the first time. It is really hard for a patient to hear things for the first time during the overwhelming period post op."
> - "I believe that patients and patients' families are more knowledgeable regarding on what they need to do and what they expect during hospitalization post operatively."

high mean scores for all areas of postoperative care (**Fig. 3**). When asked about their ability to participate in postoperative care after viewing the preoperative DVD, scores indicated patients thought that they were able to participate or able to participate a great deal in all areas (**Fig. 4**). Patients reported that the preoperative DVD was effective overall in preparing them and their family members for postoperative care activities. One patient commented that "it was extremely helpful to be able to take the DVD home." Another patient reportedly "had one long surgery at UCLA in January of 2007" and further stated, "this DVD was not available at the time…I have another longer surgery in September of 2007, and this has been helpful."

DISCUSSION

Elevated scores for knowledge, engagement, and understanding may be attributable to the incorporation of the DVD in the preoperative teaching. A quality instructional media product was developed, implemented, and found to be effective in increasing preoperative knowledge and preparedness of patients and their families. Nurses

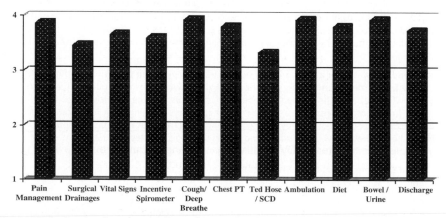

Fig. 3. Mean levels of understanding of postoperative care activities reported by patients surveyed after the intervention. PT, physiotherapy.

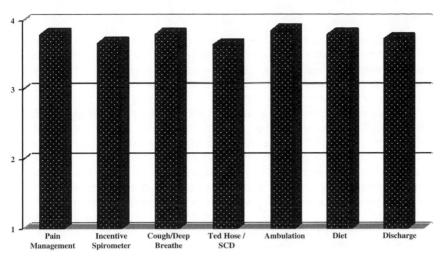

Fig. 4. Mean levels of ability to participate in postoperative care activities reported by patients surveyed after the intervention.

reported higher levels of knowledge and engagement of patients and their families related to postoperative activities. The supposition is that use of the DVD would increase knowledge and provide useful information to enhance the level of involvement of patients in their postoperative activities. The accessibility of information about postoperative care provided opportunities for viewing by the patient and family members. This format enabled patients to review the information numerous times at their own pace. It is not known whether this format influenced outcomes, such as length of stay. It is assumed, however, that the more active patients are in their own care, the more likely they are to progress toward short-term and long-term goals.

This important evidence-based practice project emphasized the value of incorporating DVDs as a part of the preoperative teaching process. The findings delineate the necessity for providing patient-specific postoperative care instruction before patients undergo thoracic surgery. "The goal of patient teaching is to improve patients' understanding of their disease process and the operation that they are about to experience, with the goal of enlisting their active participation in the healing process."[2] This goal is best reached through the collaborative efforts of the health care providers involved in the patients' care. In turn, an eager and well-informed patient can become a participating member of the health care team.[2]

The development of the preoperative DVD was based on existing evidence-based literature and the needs of patients after thoracic surgery. As a result, the findings of this project and the DVD may be limited in generalizability to a small sample of patients and nurses in acute thoracic surgical settings. The magnitude of the effect of the intervention may be too small to detect. Replication of this study with a larger sample size is warranted. A potential effect of time is related to the nurse and patient survey assessments after the DVD intervention. Changing the system was a challenge. The clinic, which is located offsite, lacks an infrastructure to ensure the distribution of preoperative teaching and educational materials. The outcomes of this project clearly delineate the benefits of implementing a preoperative DVD in an effort to meet postoperative care goals, however. This project enhanced thoracic surgical patients' knowledge of, engagement in, and understanding of their postoperative care activities.

SUMMARY

Patients' outcomes were improved by changing the system so that patients were consistently provided with a preoperative instructional DVD. The connection between the patient's postoperative experience and preoperative teaching is intimately linked. This evidence-based project clearly demonstrates that for patients who have had thoracic surgery, and perhaps patients in other acute surgical settings, the need for information about their postoperative care and potential complications obligates health care providers to ensure that patients receive the information they need to engage in their care. Health care practitioners should consider providing this information in a DVD format to supplement verbal and written instruction. A DVD provides an effective and efficient method of distributing important postoperative care information and may enhance patients' ability to recall key aspects of their preoperative instruction. In turn, patients are well equipped to exert confidence and empowered control over their performance of clinically relevant activities after surgery. Perhaps the greatest advantage is the patient's ability to access and view the instructional DVD easily within the confines of his or her home as opposed to a medical office or hospital room.

ACKNOWLEDGMENTS

The authors thank the thoracic surgeons (Drs. Cameron, Lee, Maish, and Maharaja) and Martha Martinez for their generous support. They also thank the DVD production crew, particularly Nancy Williams and Brian Williams, for their professional and understanding work. Finally, they thank to the patients and clinical staff in the medical observation unit who generously provided their time and experience.

REFERENCES

1. Bernier MJ, Sanares DC, Owen SV, et al. Preoperative teaching received and valued in a day surgery setting. AORN J 2003;77(3):563–72, 575–8, 581–2.
2. Whyte RI, Grant PD. Preoperative patient education in thoracic surgery. Thorac Surg Clin 2005;15(2):195–201.
3. Lewis C, Gunta K, Wong D. Patient knowledge, behavior, and satisfaction with the use of a preoperative DVD. Orthop Nurs 2002;21(6):41–3.
4. Oetker-Black SL, Jones S, Estok P, et al. Preoperative teaching and hysterectomy outcomes. AORN J 2003;77(6):1215–8, 1221–31.
5. Brumfield VC, Kee CC, Johnson JY. Preoperative patient teaching in ambulatory surgery settings. AORN J 1996;64(6):941–6, 948, 951–2.
6. Doering LV, McGuire AW, Rourke D. Recovering from cardiac surgery: what patients want you to know. Am J Crit Care 2002;11(4):333–43.
7. Johansson K, Nuutila L, Virtanen H, et al. Preoperative education for orthopaedic patients: systematic review. J Adv Nurs 2005;50(2):212–23.
8. Evrard S, Mathoulin-Pelissier S, Larrue C, et al. Evaluation of a preoperative multimedia information program in surgical oncology. Eur J Surg Oncol 2005; 31(1):106–10.
9. Shaban M, Salsali M, Kamali P, et al. Assessment the effects of respiratory exercise education in acute respiratory complication and the length of patient hospitalization, for undergoing coronary artery by-pass surgery in Kermanshah Emam Ali Hospital. HAYAT: J Faculty Nurs Midwifery 2002; 15:12–20 [in persian]. Available at: http://journals.tums.ac.ir/abs.aspx?org_id=59&culture_var=en&journal_id=10&segment=fa&issue_id=66&manuscript_id=577.

10. Stern C, Lockwood C. Knowledge retention from preoperative patient information. Int J Evidence-Based Healthcare 2005;3(3):45–63 Available at: http://www3. interscience.wiley.com/journal/118719400/abstract.
11. Doering S, Katzlberger F, Rumpold G, et al. Videotape preparation of patients before hip replacement surgery reduces stress. Psychosom Med 2000;62(3): 365–73.
12. Devine EC, Cook TD. A meta-analytic analysis of effects of psychoeducational interventions on length of postsurgical hospital stay. Nurs Res 1983;32(5):267–74.
13. Yount S, Schoessler M. A description of patient and nurse perceptions of preoperative teaching. J Post Anesth Nurs 1991;6(1):17–25.
14. Fitzpatrick E, Hyde A. Nurse-related factors in the delivery of preoperative patient education. J Clin Nurs 2006;15(6):671–7.
15. Hathaway D. Effect of preoperative instruction on postoperative outcomes: a meta-analysis. Nurs Res 1986;35(5):269–75 [editorial].
16. Thomas R, Deary A, Kaminski E, et al. Patients' preferences for video cassette recorded information: effect of age, sex and ethnic group. Eur J Cancer Care (Engl) 1999;8(2):83–6.
17. Titler MG, Kleiber C, Steelman VJ, et al. The Iowa model of evidence-based practice to promote quality care. Crit Care Nurs Clin North Am 2001;13(4): 497–509.

The Clinical Scholar Model: Evidence-Based Practice at the Bedside

Cynthia Honess, RN, MSN, CCRN, ACNS-BC[a],*, Paulette Gallant, RN, MSN, CNL[b],
Kathleen Keane, RN, BSN, CCRN[c]

KEYWORDS

- Evidence-based practice • Staff nurse
- Clinical scholar • Clinical scholar model
- Bedside evidence-based practice

THE CLINICAL SCHOLAR MODEL: EVIDENCE-BASED PRACTICE AT THE POINT OF CARE

The innovative design of the Clinical Scholar Model[1] enables nurses to question and reflect on traditional practices at the bedside. Maine Medical Center (MMC), a tertiary care center with more than 600 beds in northern New England, used the model to support staff nurses in developing an evidence-based practice (EBP) culture. The model empowered staff nurses to be curious, reflective, and question traditional practices. The three EBP projects described here evolved from the clinical curiosity of staff nurses. Each of the projects used the Clinical Scholar Model to guide the process of identifying, implementing, and evaluating clinical practice changes and outcomes. These projects illustrate how staff nurses use their critical thinking skills to observe, analyze, and synthesize evidence and determine its applicability to the clinical practice setting.

REDUCING THE LENGTH OF BED REST FOLLOWING A CARDIAC CATHETERIZATION OR PERCUTANEOUS CORONARY INTERVENTION

A core group of cardiology nurses used the Clinical Scholar Model as a framework to identify issues surrounding the optimal duration of bed rest for patients following a cardiac catheterization or percutaneous coronary intervention (PCI). The time the nurses spent on this project and attending the Clinical Scholar Program workshops to guide learning of EBP was supported by the nursing director.

---

[a] Center for Clinical and Professional Development, Department of Nursing, Maine Medical Center, 22 Bramhall Street, Portland, ME 04102-3175, USA
[b] Maine Medical Center, Richards 1, 22 Bramhall Street, Portland, ME 04102-3175, USA
[c] Cardiothoracic Intensive Care Unit, Maine Medical Center, 22 Bramhall Street, Portland, ME 04102-3175, USA
* Corresponding author.
E-mail address: honesc@mmc.org (C. Honess).

Nurs Clin N Am 44 (2009) 117–130
doi:10.1016/j.cnur.2008.10.004
0029-6465/08/$ – see front matter © 2009 Elsevier Inc. All rights reserved.

The optimal duration of bed rest following a cardiac catheterization or PCI is not known. Duration of bed rest postprocedure may vary from as little as 2 hours to as much as 12 hours. Maintaining bed rest is an effort to avoid complications at the vascular entry point for the procedure, which usually is the femoral artery and/or vein. Vascular complications range from bleeding at the femoral access site, hematomas of varying sizes, arterial-venous fistula, and pseudoaneurysms.[2]

Potential discomforts arise for the patient remaining on bed rest for any length of time. These discomforts include inability to flex the leg in the femoral area on the procedural side, head of the bed elevated to only 30°, and log rolling from side to side. Back and leg pain may occur related to the inability to move freely in bed or to have the head of bed elevated. Bed rest also can present problems in urinary elimination because of the change in urination habits. These issues are related significantly to patient and family satisfaction with the hospital stay and to hospitalization costs associated with pain medications, urinary catheters, and nursing care time.

Approximately 2000 patients per year experience a cardiac catheterization or PCI at MMC, and traditionally these patients remained on bed rest for 6 hours. Patients and family are the primary stakeholders in this practice, but other stakeholders include staff nurses, physicians, and nursing administrators. Garnering support from all the stakeholders was an important first step in examining the current practice regarding the duration of bed rest and in exploring the feasibility and safety of decreasing the duration of bed rest to 4 hours. For patients and families, the benefits of reducing the duration of bed rest include early ambulation, a potential decrease in pain medication usage, and adequate elimination.

The nursing staff, as stakeholders in reducing the length of postprocedure bed rest, saw an opportunity to change practice using the latest evidence and as an opportunity to improved documentation. A new postprocedure documentation tool including specific features addressing assessments for the development vascular complications over time was developed to introduce and implement this practice change.

Nursing administrators are involved in examining the feasibility of proposals for practice changes. Presenting the cost benefits of a shorter duration of bed rest to nursing administrators helped gain their support. The potential cost savings would be realized in reduced needs for analgesia and assistive equipment and shorter patient stay.

Gaining support from physician stakeholders involved multiple presentations of the results of synthesized research studies with components that paralleled the practices for these cardiac procedures at MMC. The physicians were especially concerned with the risks of vascular complications. Synthesis of the primary external evidence showed that the duration of bed rest could be reduced without increasing vascular complications.

Search and Analysis of the External Evidence

A literature search was conducted in MEDline and the Cumulative Index of Nursing and Allied Health Literature (CINAHL) using the keywords "cardiac procedures," "bed rest duration," "amounts of anticoagulation," "early ambulation," "and vascular complications." Thirty research studies were found; five studies included the variables of interest.

The five studies were critiqued using a research critique table.[3] Three of the studies were randomized, controlled trials, and two were quasi-experimental. Variables of interest included bed rest duration of 2 to 6 hours,[2,4–7] femoral access sheath dwell time of approximately zero to 6 hours following the procedure,[2,4–7] a femoral sheath size of 6 to 8 F,[2,4–7] and varying amounts of anticoagulant administered during selected cardiac procedures.[2,4–7] All studies evaluated were of acceptable quality.

Synthesizing the Internal and External Evidence

Following critique of the studies, four tables based on the variables of interest were developed to synthesize and compare the results in each of the five studies. **Table 1** is an example of a single synthesis table based on length of bed rest. Each table had the same column headings, and findings were compared with current practices within the institution.

Decreasing the length of bed rest from 6 to 4 hours without increasing vascular complications was the major goal of this evidence-based project. The studies most closely paralleling the practices at MMC were those that compared results in a control group remaining in bed for 6 hours and an interventional group that remained in bed for 4 hours. The other synthesis tables tabulated vascular complications incorporating the other variables of sheath dwell time, sheath size, and anticoagulation.

The rate of vascular complications following a cardiac catheterization or PCI was low at MMC. Events considered as complications included bleeding, hematoma, and arterial-venous fistula developing during sheath removal or at some point during bed rest. These complications were considered as internal evidence in the result of decreasing bed rest from 6 to 4 hours. External evidence[2,4–7] provided an overall complication rate of 6% related to bleeding and hematoma, higher than the current complication rate MMC.

As key stakeholders in this project, the physicians were concerned about a possible increase in vascular complications. The synthesis tables demonstrating the strength of the evidence for reducing bed rest after sheath removal from 6 hours to 4 hours convinced the physicians that the practice change would not increase the potential for risk or harm. After reviewing the framework of the Clinical Scholar Model, the cardiology team gave the project their support.

A proposal to move ahead with this EBP was drafted. The draft was based on strength of the evidence from the research studies regarding vascular complications following a reduction of bed rest from 6 to 4 hours. The provisions for bed rest were prescribed by physicians through an order set for postcardiac catheterization or PCI care.

Implementing and Evaluating: A Pilot Study

A pilot study for bed rest duration was planned to test this practice change and to assess the rate of vascular complications. As bedside clinicians, nursing staff were valuable stakeholders in the implementation and monitoring of this practice change. The cardiac interventional department identified as the pilot unit was a demanding area for nursing care. The nursing staff had been removing femoral access sheaths and establishing hemostasis in the procedural area for the past 5 years and was expert in assessing the presence of vascular complications. Their participation was needed to implement the change and successfully decrease the duration of bed rest.

A postprocedure documentation tool was developed to incorporate assessment of the femoral access site and other components that might potentiate a vascular complication. The first assessment served as a baseline for the access site condition. An area for treatment of a vascular complication was included; the designated methods for achieving hemostasis were manual compression or the use of a mechanical device. Vital signs and further assessments were entered on the documentation tool at regular intervals. The countdown to ambulation began when the femoral access sheath was removed, based on the activated clotting time being within the designated

Table 1
Length of bed rest

First Author[ref]	Sample Research Design	Independent Variable/ Intervention	Dependent Variable Outcome	Significant Results	Limitations/Gaps	Generalizability (AHRQ Levels of Evidence)
Vlasic W, et al[2]	Randomized, controlled trial N = 299 n = 99: 2 hr BR n = 99: 4 hr BR n = 101: 6 hr BR	BR: 2, 4, or 6 hr	Vascular complications Major: transfusion, surgical repair, ultrasound guided compression, prolonged hospital stay Minor: requiring site compression, hematoma < 5 × 5 cm, bleeding (soaking two 4 × 4 inch gauzes)	2-hr group 3% hematoma 4% rebleeding 1% pseudoaneurysm and surgical repair 4-hr group 6% hematoma 3% rebleeding 6-hr group 5% hematoma 2% rebleeding	Trial became unblinded after hemostasis	Yes (A)
Keeling A, et al[4]	Randomized, controlled trial N = 71 Experimental group: n = 51: 4 hr BR Control group: n = 20: 6 hr BR	4 hr of bed rest versus 6 hr of bed rest	Vascular complications	4-hr group 98% without complication. One patient had a small amount of oozing after multiple procedures and ACT > 200 at the time of sheath pull.	Incomplete data collection because of inability to place patients in the control group: doctors ordered 4 hr of bed rest	Yes (B)
Koch K, et al[5]	Descriptive N = 300 patients	2 hr bed rest	Vascular complications Bleeding at ambulation Late bleeding: ambulation to 48 hr Hematoma > 5 × 5 cm Arterial-venous fistula Pseudoaneurysm	2-hr group 1.7% bleeding at ambulation 3% hematoma > 5 × 5 cm No late bleeding	Patients taking oral anticoagulants or heparin before the procedure were excluded Use of compression bandage	No (B)

Koch K, et al[6]	Quasi-experimental N = 830 n = 420: 4 hr BR n = 410: BR overnight	Experimental group = 4 hr of bed rest Control group = Bedrest overnight	Vascular complications Bleeding at ambulation Late bleeding: ambulation to 48 hr Hematoma > 5 × 5 cm Arterial-venous fistula Pseudoaneurysm	4-hr group: 2.3% all complications 4-hr to overnight group: 2.2% all complications	Patients taking oral anticoagulants or heparin before the procedure were excluded Non randomized use of compression bandage	No (B)
Bogart M, et al[7]	Randomized, controlled trial N = 200 Experimental: n = 100: 4 hr BR Control: n = 100: 6 hr BR	Experimental group: 4 hr BR Control group: 6 hr BR	Vascular complications Rebleeding Hematoma Arteriovenous fistula Pseudoaneurysm Limb ischemia Thrombosis of femoral artery Hematoma: Small (< 5 cm) Medium (6–10 cm) Large (> 10 cm)	4 hr group: 1% small hematoma 6-hr group: 2% rebleeding 1% pseudoaneurysm	After cardiac catherization, 79% of patients in the experimental group and 71% of patients in the control group received heparin during the procedure	Yes (B)

Abbreviations: ACT, active clotting time; AGCHR, Agency for Health care and Research Quality; BR, bed rest.

range. The method for compression of the femoral access site following sheath removal was identified on the form. The final assessment was an observation of the femoral access site 15 minutes after initiating activity. Exclusions to ambulation at 4 hours were hypertension, sedation, and the development of bleeding or hematoma during bed rest. The postprocedure documentation tool was used to collect quality improvement data at different points in time as well as to provide assessment guidelines.

One of the goals of this EBP project was the absence of vascular complications when bed rest was reduced. After pilot testing for 6 months, there had been no increase in vascular complications. This outcome was communicated to physicians and nursing through cardiology staff and nursing staff meetings. Order sets for postcardiac procedural care were adapted to reflect the 4 hours of bed rest.

Using the framework of the Clinical Scholar Model as a guide, this nurse workgroup identified a clinical practice issue and the evidence needed to support a successful practice change after PCI. It was estimated that over a 1-month period this change in practice resulted in a saving of 300 hours of nursing time, time that could be spent providing patient education and other nursing care. Audits for the development of vascular complication continue with the postprocedure record.

Dissemination

The core group of cardiology nurses involved in this EBP project shared their reflections on the Clinical Scholar Model and this project with their colleagues at the hospital and at national and international research conferences. The practice of reduced bed rest is sustained by the change in order sets and the postprocedure record. Nursing staff directly sustain the practice of reduced bed rest following a cardiac catheterization or PCI through efforts to avoid vascular complications while maintaining patient comfort.

REDUCING POSTOPERATIVE NAUSEA AND VOMITING IN PATIENTS UNDERGOING OPEN-HEART SURGERY

The following project illustrates using the Clinical Scholar Model in a different setting at MMC, the cardiothoracic ICU (CTICU). Bedside nurses are astute observers of patients' experiences and responses in health and illness. As a part of their critical thinking processes, staff nurses continuously ask questions about their practice and reflect on the efficacy of their interventions. The richness of the bedside nursing practice and the questions generated are fertile ground for beginning the process of changing nursing practice based on supporting evidence.

Staff nurses in the CTICU observed that many of their patients experienced postoperative nausea and/or vomiting (PONV) during the recovery period. The nurses questioned the current practice protocol. Some of the questions they asked were

Is treatment of PONV enough?
Should we be doing more to prevent PONV?
Is our current rescue treatment with ondansetron adequate?
What are the most efficacious pharmacologic measures for prevention and treatment of PONV?
Are there nonpharmacologic treatments for PONV?

A practice-driven clinical question was formulated: "Is the current protocol we use to treat postoperative nausea and vomiting evidence based?" Three staff nurses formed a core nurse workgroup and explored this question. These nurses already were attending the workshops in the Clinical Scholar Program, and the time they spent at the workshops and working on the project was supported by the CTICU nursing director.

Search and Analysis of the External Evidence

The nurse workgroup began with a search for external evidence. Prevalence studies of PONV in patients undergoing open-heart surgery (OHS) showed that this clinical issue was a common problem in this population.[8] The focus of the search turned to the efficacy of pharmacologic treatment strategies for PONV. The challenges of the search became apparent when simple searches in multiples databases revealed thousands of individual articles on various aspects of treatment and prevention of PONV. In this case, there was substantial external evidence, and the primary challenge was how to sift through and synthesize the information relevant to the clinical question.

The Clinical Scholar workshops supported the nurse workgroup in exploring the literature and learning about the levels of evidence that supported practice change. With a well-designed approach[9] to grading the evidence, it became clear that there were meta-analyses, as well as individual studies, that discussed the treatment and prevention of PONV. Unlike the Agency for Health care and Research Quality level of evidence table used in the previous example, the levels of evidence used to grade the reviewed evidence included well-designed quantitative studies, meta-analyses, qualitative research, quality improvement data, and expert opinion. Additional evidence in the form of consensus clinical guidelines was reviewed by the core nurse workgroup. The use of these broad sources of evidence to examine the clinical question strengthened the basis with which they approached the clinical issue[10] and contributed with an approach that was patient centered.

Recognizing the utility of a guideline in summarizing clinical information, the nurse workgroup identified a clinical guideline[11] that addressed the key issues identified in their meetings. They critiqued the guideline using a framework suggested by Brown[12] and gained insight into an overview of the process for addressing PONV in a clinical setting. The evidence reviewed demonstrated that the process of preventing and treating PONV was well studied and well understood. Risk-assessment studies[13,14] indicated that patients after OHS were at risk for PONV because of a variety of factors, including the length of the surgery and the use of postoperative narcotics. With use of the guideline, it also became clear that prophylaxis involves treatment of the patient before induction of anesthetic as well as treatment in the postoperative phase. The nurse workgroup realized anesthesiologists would be key stakeholders in the project, and they invited a physician colleague to join the project. The anesthesiologist brought important contributions to the workgroup through his knowledge of individual studies[15] that pertained to the efficacy of steroids for PONV in the OHS population. Another stakeholder who joined the core workgroup was a pharmacist dedicated to the ICU setting; his knowledge of the drug therapies and formulary options at MMC was very helpful. Other key stakeholders included the nursing director of the unit, the CTICU staff nurses who implemented a pilot of the project, the cardiothoracic surgeons, and their physician assistants. Building consensus on recognizing the need for EBP change involved the entire culture of the CTICU.

Synthesizing the Internal and External Evidence

The nurse workgroup saw that PONV was common in their postoperative patients, so they conducted a preliminary 2-week chart audit on the OHS cases. Using antiemetic usage as a flag for PONV, they noted that 50% of patients required treatment for PONV in the first 3 days after surgery. Quality-improvement audits gathered from patients before discharge indicated that patients reported nausea as a major problem postoperatively. This site-specific internal evidence validated the concerns of the staff nurses and supported the need for further exploration of the clinical question.

The external evidence[11] indicated that prevention of PONV should begin for patients before induction of anesthesia via the administration of dexamethasone. Another prophylactic dose of antiemetic, ondansetron, should be administered in the immediate postoperative period. Further rescue therapy for treatment of breakthrough PONV followed a key principle called "multimodal treatment": that is, should breakthrough PONV occur, it should be treated with a pharmacologic agent with a mechanism of action different from that of the previously used agents. For this reason, prochlorperazine was added to the protocol for treatment of breakthrough PONV.

Implementation and Evaluation

Through a review of the evidence and interdisciplinary collaboration with representatives from anesthesia and pharmacy, a new evidence-based protocol was developed for preventing and treating patients experiencing PONV after OHS. Nurses and physicians from the CTICU were invited to review the proposed changes and share their concerns. The proposal for change was submitted to and reviewed by the hospital's institutional review board. Detailed baseline data before protocol implementation provided a basis of comparison for evaluating the protocol's efficacy. The use of this new protocol and analysis of data before and after protocol implementation showed that patients experienced a significant decrease in the incidence and prevalence of PONV in the CTICU. Implementation of the protocol resulted in a 50% overall reduction in patient episodes of PONV from the day of surgery to 4 days after surgery. The protocol was most effective in reducing PONV on the day of surgery and on postoperative day one. Cost analysis showed that the new protocol did not increase the amount of ondansetron used and provided better patient outcomes.

Dissemination

The nurse workgroup involved in this study shared its findings at the unit and hospital level and at national and international conferences. Along with its findings, it proposed suggestions to enhance project sustainability. These suggestions included embedding the data collection and data analysis of the protocol into systems already in place in the clinical microsystem, thereby enhancing the ability continually to review and improve delivery at the point of care.

The systematic process of studying this clinical question using the Clinical Scholar Model provided these clinical scholars with answers as well as even more questions about the clinical experiences of their patients. The protocol developed was effective in treating early-onset PONV, but after OHS many patients also experience later-onset PONV or PONV that persisted throughout their hospital stay. More research in this area is needed to understand the effectiveness of treatments and interventions. In addition, as new therapies evolve, the evidence supporting practice will change. The challenge for clinical scholars is to review and re-evaluate the evidence as it is disseminated; clinical knowledge is evolving at a pace that brings a wealth of both quantitative and qualitative knowledge to the bedside.

IMPROVING GLYCEMIC CONTROL IN AN OPEN-HEART SURGERY PROGRAM

For several years, the Clinical Scholar Model has been used as a format for identifying an issue, assessing internal and external evidence, synthesizing the evidence, implementing and evaluating a change in practice, and disseminating the results in the step-down (intermediate care) unit for patients after OHS. In addition to dissemination, an interdisciplinary team recently evaluated the sustainability of a practice change and subsequent outcomes. In 2004A the cardiothoracic surgical team at MMC instituted a continuous insulin infusion (CII) protocol in the OHS population, but adherence to the CII protocol (ie, a blood glucose goal of 110 mg/dL in the ICU patients and 150 mg/dL for patients in the step-down unit) had never been evaluated. Also, it had not been determined whether the rates of deep sternal wound infection (DSWI) had been reduced after implementation of the CII protocol.

Search and Analysis of the External Evidence

This protocol was based on the research studies conducted by Furnary,[16–18] which showed that using a CII for 72 hours postoperatively on all patients undergoing heart surgery reduced DSWI and mortality. Before Furnary's[16–18] studies, only diabetics were treated with insulin, and the insulin usually was given subcutaneously. Van Den Berghe's[19] research on patients in intensive care concluded that patients who had abnormal glucose tests had a much higher risk of infection and mortality. In addition, in their position statement the American College of Endocrinology[20] recommended a blood glucose of 110 mg/dL or below be maintained for all patients in surgical intensive care.

Synthesizing the External and Internal Evidence

Based on the evidence supporting the use of CII in patients undergoing heart surgery, the cardiothoracic team developed a protocol based on the work of Furnary.[18] The protocol was developed and initiated in both the CTICU and the step-down unit. The protocol was initiated upon the patient's arrival at the ICU, and it was continued for 96 hours postoperatively. The nursing staff, the doctors, and the physician assistants received minimal education on the use of the protocol, and the protocol was received with skepticism and uneasiness related to the fear of hypoglycemia. Also, there was no plan for an evaluation of the success or failure of the protocol. The only data point collected was the incidence of DSWI, which remained unchanged at 3%. The clinicians' prevailing perception was that the use of the CII would guarantee good glucose control. Random checks of glucose levels in the cardiac surgery population showed glucose levels consistently were above 200 mg/dL, levels that were alarming. In addition, the CII protocol was not followed in either the ICU or the step-down unit.

Implementation and Evaluation

The initial goal of the glucose project was to determine nurses' adherence to the CII protocol. The original team members included a staff nurse, a physician assistant, and a physician. As the glycemic control project progressed, other team members were added to obtain their expertise; at various times, the team included a dietician, staff nurses, data analysts, medical students, a clinical nurse specialist, perfusionists, and anesthesiologists.

In the initial glycemic control protocol, the target glucose level was 110 mg/dL or less in the CTICU and 150 mg/dL or less in the step-down unit, based on evidence from the work of Furnary[16–18] and Van den Berghe.[19] As part of the ongoing quality improvement program, a data collection tool was developed and approved by the MMC institutional review board that included the name, age, and gender of the patient; the procedure performed; the patient's height, weight, and fasting blood sugar; diagnosis of diabetes; transfusion of blood products; all glucose recordings; and treatment for 96 hours. Blood product information was collected because there is ongoing evidence that patients undergoing heart surgery who receive blood products are at increased risk for mortality and infection.[21] Following completion of each phase of the glycemic control project, the data analyst for the Northern New England Cardiovascular Disease Study Group provided additional information on length of stay, DSWI, and mortality.

Body mass index (BMI) and hemoglobin A1c were added as data points in subsequent phases. BMI is a more definitive measure of obesity than height and weight. Abnormal BMIs in patients correlate with higher glucose levels even when the patients do not have a diagnosis of diabetes.[22,23] Hemoglobin A1c was added in the preoperative order set for all patients undergoing heart surgery to give the practitioner information about previous control of a patient's diabetes and/or to indicate a need for further testing for diabetes if the preoperative test was abnormal.[24,25] In previous studies, the risk for infection was highest in the first 72 hours following surgery.[16–18] The team decided to collect data on 150 patients, approximately one eighth of the annual adult heart surgery population. A proposal was developed and sent to the institutional review board for review and approval. After approval, data were collected on 157 consecutive patients undergoing heart surgery.

Evaluation of the Glycemic Control Project: Phase One

Findings from the first phase showed that the mean glucose levels ranged from 128 to 158 mg/dL in the first 96 hours postoperatively, the CII protocol was stopped prematurely in the first 24 hours postoperatively, and the full CII protocol was not followed. In addition, the DSWI rate during the 3 months of the glycemic study was 3.3%, as compared with a target rate of less than 1%. As a result of these findings, the CII protocol was revised, and intensive education on diabetes and hyperglycemia was presented to the nurses in the critical care and step-down units, the physician assistants, and cardiothoracic physicians. It was hypothesized that education would increase both knowledge and comfort level with the CII protocol. The education was done both formally through short educational sessions and informally through discussions on glucose control and use of the protocol. Education was accomplished by physicians, a physician assistant, a unit-based educator, and a diabetic clinical nurse specialist. Daily discussions with nurses, physicians, and physician assistants focused on efforts for reducing DSWI through the implementation of good glycemic control. This approach with education conducted by a team was successful in reaching coworkers.

Revisions, Implementation, and Monitoring: Phase Two

In phase two, the target glucose range for patients in the critical care and the step-down units was increased from 110 mg/dL in the ICU and 150 mg/dL in the step-down unit to 150 mg/dL in both units. This change was made to increase the comfort level of the heart surgery team with a future goal of decreasing the upper limit of glucose to 120 mg/dL.

Many things happened during the second phase of this project. In response to multiple complaints about the three-page length of the CII protocol, three medical students developed a nomogram. This user-friendly, color-coded one-page format was well received by nurses, physician assistants, and doctors and has continued to be used with minor changes based on the findings during the subsequent phases of the glycemic control project. During this second phase, patients remained on the CII protocol for 96 hours. Phase two mean glucose levels from admission to the operating room to 96 hours postoperatively were found to be in the range of 124 to140 mg/dL. No DSWI occurred during 6 months. One of the findings from phase two was the number of abnormal glucose levels in both the known and unknown diabetic population at the 96-hour mark: 25% of the patients were prediabetic or new type 2 diabetics with previously undiagnosed diabetes. This finding created a new dilemma, because most of these patients would be discharged within 24 to 48 hours.

A New Dilemma With a Creative Solution

There were ongoing discussions among physicians, nurses, and physician assistants about how to solve the new problems that arose from the findings in the glucose study. As a result, a team met with to find a solution that (1) would not increase length of stay but would provide a safety net for the patient and (2) would not increase the workload of the staff nurse. A collaborative team including dieticians, dietary aides, nurses, physicians, a diabetic nurse specialist, Lifescan representatives, a laboratory representative, and physician assistants convened to look at both the dietary and discharge needs of the patients. Providing more dietary options for patients and providing new diabetics with a free glucometer and educational materials were two of the decisions made by this collaborative group. In addition, information about poorly controlled diabetics and new diabetics was sent to the patients' primary care physicians.

Revisions, Implementation, and Monitoring: Phase Three

Following minor revisions in the nomogram for the CII protocol and the development of an insulin infusion start chart to differentiate dose amounts depending on a patient's blood glucose nadir, phase three of the glucose project was conducted. In addition to determining compliance with the CII protocol, data for the discharge plan were collected for the newly diagnosed and poorly controlled diabetics.

During phase three data collection, the cardiothoracic team found several alarming issues:

1. An increase in leg infections
2. No change in mediastinitis or mortality rates
3. Lack of standardization for patients transitioning off the CII protocol
4. Several incidences of hypoglycemia in discharged patients, with one patient readmitted to the hospital with seizures

These findings led to three changes: re-education of nurses about the importance of glucose control, development of a transition protocol to be used when the CII protocol is discontinued, and a preoperative order for hemoglobin A1c for all patients undergoing cardiac surgery.

Changes in practice were made within 1 month. Delays in surgery that occurred because of double-digit hemoglobin A1c and abnormal glucose levels resulted in patients being treated aggressively to bring glucose levels down to a normal level before surgery. Based on the results from Funary's research,[16–18] the risk for DSWI from hyperglycemia diminished by postoperative day three. Because of these findings at the end of phase three of the study, the team decided to discontinue the CII protocol on the morning of postoperative day three.

Plans for Phase Four

Furnary[22] used a CII tight glycemic protocol in the first 72 hours postoperatively when patients were at highest risk for DSWI. Based on Funary's findings, the team decided to discontinue the CII protocol on the morning of postoperative day three. A transition protocol was developed for use when the CII protocol was discontinued: to standardize the approach for glucose levels above 150 mg/dL, short-acting insulin was administered subcutaneously for correctional coverage. In addition, patients who had a previous diagnosis of diabetes resumed their preoperative regimen on the evening of postoperative day two or on the morning of postoperative day three. The exceptions to this approach were patients who were taking Metformin Hcl and had an elevated creatinine level, diabetic patients who were poorly controlled, and newly diagnosed diabetics. The transition protocol will be evaluated in phase four of the hyperglycemia project.

The cardiothoracic team is aware that ongoing assessment of the CII protocol is needed to reduce each patient's risk for mortality and morbidity following cardiac surgery. In addition to reducing the DSWI rate, the team has developed a consistent approach for glycemic control in the heart surgery population.

Interdisciplinary Respect and Collaboration

The greatest accomplishment to date has been the collaboration among all team members in identifying problems or issues involving the cardiothoracic population. This interdisciplinary team allows all voices to be heard in a nonpunitive atmosphere. This collaborative model has thrived and been sustained for 3 years with the ultimate goal of providing patients with best possible outcomes. The same collaborative approach has been used to implement oral care, prevent pressure ulcers, improve wound care, and develop a ventricular assist device protocol. Informal bi-weekly 30-minute meetings are held to identify any issues within the cardiothoracic patient population and/or issues with staff relationships. Doctors, nurses, physician assistants, management, nursing assistants, and other disciplines are invited to attend. The relationship among the team members filters to the daily work environment, where communication is key to providing the best possible outcomes for patients. Opinions about a patient's condition are heard, and complications are averted because of this unique model. This collaborative model now is being used to implement glycemic control in all inpatient areas throughout the hospital.

SUMMARY

Using the Clinical Scholar Model, staff nurses can evaluate the evidence supporting clinical practice at the point of care. Following the model through the steps was easy for a novice bedside researcher. This model gave clinical staff nurses an avenue for conducting nursing research and implementing evidence-based changes that are meaningful in their daily practice. In addition, the process increased collaborative conversations among health care providers, patients, and families about evidence-based care.

The Clinical Scholar Model serves as an effective guide for investigating and implementing EBP change at the bedside. It assists in identifying problems and issues, the key stakeholders, and the need for change in practice. These three projects, although identifying different clinical issues, followed the format of the Clinical Scholar Model. The completed projects improved patient outcomes. These projects illustrate some real-life examples of bringing this process to the clinical setting and of using the Clinical Scholar Model in practice.

ACKNOWLEDGMENTS

C.H. acknowledges the invaluable assistance of Trudy Kent, RN, BSN, Sue Chenoweth, RN, BSN, and Sara Kovacs RN, BSN. K.K. acknowledges the invaluable assistance of Bethany Drabik, RN, BSN, CCRN, and Anne Marie Gray, RN, BSN, CCRN.

REFERENCES

1. Schultz A. Origins and aspirations: conceiving the clinical scholar model. Excellence in Nursing Knowledge 2005;1–4 [online publication].
2. Vlasic W, Almond D, Massel D, et al. Reducing bed rest following arterial puncture for coronary interventional procedures. J Invasive Cardiol 2001;13:788–92 A.
3. Gallant P. Analysis: what's all the speak about critique? Excellence in Nursing Knowledge 2005;1–5 [online publication].
4. Keeling A, Fisher C, Haugh K, et al. Reducing time in bed after percutaneous transluminal coronary angioplasty. Am J Crit Care 2000;9:185–7 B.
5. Koch K, Piek J, de Winter R, et al. 2Hr ambulation after PCI with a 6 F guiding catheter and low dose heparin. Heart 1999;81:53–6 B.
6. Koch K, Piek J, de Winter R, et al. Early ambulation after coronary angioplasty and stenting with 6F guiding catheters and low dose heparin. Am J Cardiol 1997;80: 1084–6 B.
7. Bogart M, Bogart D, Rigden, et al. A prospective randomized trial of early ambulation following 8F diagnostic cardiac catheterization. Catheter Cardiovasc Interv 1999;47:175–8 B.
8. Mace L. An audit of post-operative nausea and vomiting, following cardiac surgery: scope of the problem. Nurs Crit Care 2003;8(5):187–96 B.
9. Stetler C, Brunell M, Giuliano K, et al. Evidence-based practice and the role of nursing leadership. J Nurs Adm 1998;28:45–53.
10. Rycroft-Malone J, Seers K, Titchen A, et al. What counts as evidence in evidence-based practice? J Adv Nurs 2004;47:81–90 B.
11. Gan T, Meyer T, Apfel C, et al. Consensus guidelines for managing postoperative nausea and vomiting. Anesth Analg 2003;97(1):62 B.
12. Brown SJ. Knowledge for health care practice: a guide to using research evidence. Philadelphia: W.B. Saunders Company; 1999.
13. Apfel C, Kranke P, Eberhart A. Comparison of predictive models for postoperative nausea and vomiting. Br J Anaesth 2002;88:234–40 B.
14. Koivuranta M, Laara E, Alahuhta S. A survey of postoperative nausea and vomiting. Anaesthesia 1997;52(5):443–9 B.
15. Halvorsen P, Raeder J, White PF, et al. The effect of dexamethasone on side effects after coronary revascularization procedures. Anesth Analg 2003;96:1578–83 A.
16. Zerr K, Furnary A, Grunkemeier G, et al. Glucose control lowers the risk of wound infection in diabetics after open heart operations. Ann Thorac Surg 1997;63: 353–61.
17. Furnary A, Zerr K, Grunkemeier G, et al. Continuous intravenous insulin infusion reduces the incidence of deep sternal wound infection in diabetic patients after cardiac surgery procedures. Ann Thorac Surg 1999;67:352–62.
18. Furnary A, Guangqiang G, Grunkemeier G, et al. Continuous insulin infusion reduces mortality inpatients with diabetes undergoing coronary artery bypass grafting. J Thorac Cardiovasc Surg 2003;125(5):1007–21.
19. Van den Berghe G, Wouters P, Weekers F, et al. Intensive insulin therapy in critically ill patients. N Engl J Med. 2001;345(19):1359–67.
20. American College of Endocrinology. Position statement on inpatient diabetes and metabolic control. Endocr Pract 2004;10(1):1–6.
21. Ferraris V, Ferraris S, Sibu S, et al. Perioperative blood transfusion and blood conservation in cardiac surgery: the Society of Thoracic Surgeons and the Society of Cardiovascular Anesthesiologist clinical practice guideline. Ann Thorac Surg 2007;83:S27–86.

22. Gandhi GY, Nuttall GA, Abel MD, et al. Intraoperative hyperglycemia and perioperative outcomes in cardiac surgery. Mayo Clin Proc 2005;80(7):862–6.

23. Rady MY, Johnson DJ, Bhavesh P, et al. Influence of individual characteristics on outcome of glycemic control in intensive care patients with or without diabetes mellitus. Mayo Clin Proc 2005;80(12):1558–67.

24. American Diabetes Association. Clinical practice recommendations 2008. Diabetes Care 2008;31:S38–41.

25. Dailey G. Assessing glycemic control with self-monitoring of blood glucose and hemoglobin A1c measurements. Mayo Clin Proc 2007;82(2):229–36.

Using Evidence to Improve Care for the Vulnerable Neonatal Population

Cheryl A. Lefaiver, PhD, RN[a],*, Phyllis Lawlor-Klean, RNC, MS, APN/CNS[b],
Rosanna Welling, RN, BSN, MBA[b], Jean Smith, RNC, BSN, MSN (c)[b],
Laura Waszak, RN[b], Wendy Tuzik Micek, PhD, RN[a]

KEYWORDS

- Neonatal intensive care nursing
- Evidence-based practice implementation
- Evidence-based practice facilitation
- Parental visitation • Feeding readiness

The movement of evidence-based practice (EBP) into the clinical setting has become important to ensure that patients receive the best nursing care possible. Although the need to incorporate evidence into bedside care may be apparent, there is not a magic recipe for successfully implementing the use of evidence at the bedside. This article describes practical ways to overcome barriers and facilitate the implementation of evidence through two examples in a Magnet-designated 650-bed not-for-profit teaching medical center, Advocate Christ Medical Center in Oak Lawn, IL, within the specialty care environment of a 37-bed level III co-perinatal center neonatal ICU (NICU).

Barriers to the use of research have been studied extensively. Nurses are limited mainly by inadequate time on the job to implement new ideas, a lack of awareness of research findings, and insufficient time to read research.[1–4] Consistent with the literature, a study of 336 nurses in the Advocate Christ Medical Center using the Funk BARRIERS research tool[1] identified the greatest barrier to using research as being inadequate time to read research. Open-ended comments identified several specific suggestions to facilitate the use of research: having as a standardized format to critique the literature, having results of research more available, and having assistance available to help nurses understand the results of research. Findings from the literature as well as the authors' institutional research suggest that staff nurses

[a] Advocate Christ Medical Center/Hope Children's Hospital, 4440 West 95th Street, Oak Lawn, IL 60453, USA
[b] Neonatal Intensive Care Unit, Advocate Christ Medical Center/Hope Children's Hospital, 4440 West 95th Street, Oak Lawn, IL 60453, USA
* Corresponding author.
E-mail address: Cheryl.Lefaiver@advocatehealth.com (C.A. Lefaiver).

Nurs Clin N Am 44 (2009) 131–144
doi:10.1016/j.cnur.2008.10.005
0029-6465/08/$ – see front matter © 2009 Elsevier Inc. All rights reserved.
nursing.theclinics.com

perceive the use of research as the explicit use of published research reports and expect health care organizations to bear responsibility for facilitation.

Melnyk and Fineout-Overholt[5] defined research use as the incorporation of research findings from a single study and defined EBP as a process involving the synthesis of the best available evidence, including research, clinical expertise, and patient preferences. Nurses in the clinical setting often relate to the meaning of EBP more readily than to the what they assume the meaning of the term "research" to be. Staff nurses, however, do not understand clearly the distinction between EBP and research. The assumption often is that "evidence" equals published research reports. Nurses certainly will be disenchanted if they assume that practice is founded exclusively on research, because so much of nursing practice has not been formally studied. Kitson and colleagues[6] and Rycroft-Malone and colleagues[7] challenge the assumption that evidence should rely primarily on original research. The authors propose that knowledge generated from evidence can be gained from the sources of (1) research, (2) clinical experience, (3) patients, clients, and caregivers, and (4) the local context and environment.[7] It is important for nurses to accept a broader definition of what constitutes evidence, particularly in specialty clinical areas such as the NICU where nursing research is limited. As the primary care providers within a health care environment, nurses must realize that they have influence because of their experience, interaction with patient and family, and the context of the care environment.

CLINICAL NURSING RESEARCH

Nurses practicing at the bedside often generate the best clinical questions because they are the link between research and practice. Both clinical projects described in this article originated from nursing staff who questioned current practice. The ideas were developed in response to practice issues, and broad sources of evidence were sought to guide project implementation, evaluation, and modification. Nurses are capable of developing ideas for change in practice, but the environment must be one where nurses feel safe to share their ideas and have the opportunity to explore and influence change in practice.

The health care environment is changing constantly. Staff nurses constitute the largest component of the health care delivery system and should have input about how they practice every day. McCormack and colleagues[8] described the concept of "context" as a necessary component for the integration of evidence into the practice setting. The authors likened the environmental context to the practice setting and suggested that a specific culture within the setting underpins the working of the organization. Findings from the Funk[1] BARRIERS survey substantiate the importance of the organizational culture, because nurses largely perceive elements of the setting, such as inadequate time to implement new ideas, as barriers to research facilitation. Therefore, if nurses are expected to use evidence in practice, leaders must create a culture where nurses feel encouraged and valued for their contributions.

Although an organization's culture is intangible, the availability of resources is one tangible way for nurses to see the value of the use of evidence at the bedside. Facilitation of EBP within a supportive culture depends largely on the access to and strategic use of resources. Resources such as access to a library and electronic research databases are necessary, but the right people are indispensable for the process of EBP facilitation. Skills and attributes required of an effective facilitator include being flexible, energetic, a catalyst for change, sensitive, a team builder, and a good communicator.[9] The role of EBP facilitation can be delegated to a variety of leaders in an organization. At Advocate Christ Medical Center, EBP facilitation is led strategically by the director of nursing research and is operationalized by the professional nurse researcher and the clinical nurse specialists (CNSs). Several strategies have led to the successful facilitation and implementation of EBP.

ROLE OF THE PROFESSIONAL NURSE RESEARCHER

The nurse researcher is employed full time, with 100% of services provided for the staff of the organization. A distinct advantage to having a dedicated person responsible for the facilitation of EBP is the protected time to work directly with nurses from all practice settings and at varying skill levels. Furthermore, this person participates on multiple hospital councils and provides a voice for the incorporation of evidence throughout the organization. Harvey and colleagues[9] describe the facilitator as being concerned with doing for others or enabling others. The nurse researcher in this organization facilitates by enabling others, as well as by doing for others when necessary. One-on-one meetings between the nurse researcher and nurses interested in pursuing EBP projects have been a very successful way to educate staff and monitor progress through evolution of the projects. The education can be tailored to the specific needs of the nurses working on the project, and the personal interaction helps the staff know that their project is meaningful. Naturally, individual meetings may seem an inefficient method for distributing information about EBP to the entire organization. Therefore, in addition to individual meetings with project leaders, the nurse researcher meets with various clinical teams who will be working on EBP projects and collaborates with CNSs who strengthen the message of EBP. The extension of the EBP culture is accomplished when nurses who have been involved in a practice change share their positive experiences with others. Furthermore, CNSs employed on each nursing unit reinforce the EBP culture at the unit level.

ROLE OF THE CLINICAL NURSE SPECIALIST

The second edition of the "Statement on Clinical Nurse Specialist Practice and Education" (2004) states, "The essence of CNS practice is clinical expertise based on advanced knowledge of nursing science."[10] Additionally, it states, "The context for CNS practice is the specialty. The specialty directs specific knowledge and skill acquisition; thus, the specialty area shapes the core competencies of clinical expertise."[10] These are two very powerful statements when working with a nursing staff of 140 in a specialty clinical environment. Guiding others into action can be done in many different ways, but the authors' most successful avenue has been mentoring through the use of leadership, collaboration, and consultation skills. The traditional CNS model incorporates the subroles of practitioner, educator, researcher, consultant, administrator, and change agent. As the researcher, the CNS promotes scientific inquiry by integrating relevant nursing research into practice, assists staff incorporating EBP into bedside practice, and expands the scientific base of nursing practice by participating in or conducting original clinical research. These actions assimilate within the patient/client sphere, nursing and nursing practice sphere, and the organizations and systems sphere of CNS practice competencies. All of these components are important during the evolution of an idea and throughout the actual implementation of an EBP change at the bedside.

In the Advocate Christ Medical Center, each nursing unit has a leadership dyad comprised of a manager of clinical operations (MCO) and a CNS. This leadership structure helps the facilitation of EBP, because the MCO is accountable for the management of the staff time and operational activities, and the CNS is accountable for implementation of practice modifications and professional development. The following description of two EBP changes provides some insight into the role of unit nursing leadership in helping staff implement EBP changes in the NICU. Fortunately, the NICU staff is very motivated and willing to work with their peer group, a fundamental necessity for success in the implementation of an EBP change. Change does not happen overnight. Mentoring others through change entails leadership preparation, encouragement, and candor about the repetition that usually is needed to change practice.

The motivation or desire to create change may come from various avenues. The NICU projects evolved from a different impetus, but in both circumstances support from unit nursing leadership was essential for success. The practice change in open visitation evolved from parental requests and a medical center safety initiative to include the patient in the shift report. The feeding readiness EBP project evolved from supporting two staff nurses' attendance at a professional conference regarding the subject and then allowing them to explore the use of their new knowledge. Guidance from the CNS and MCO included support of staff involvement, development of an implementation plan, and encouragement to expand the complexity of the projects. The need for assistance from the nurse researcher emerged as the projects progressed; in particular, the researcher provided guidance in submitting the feeding readiness project to the institutional review board (IRB) and assistance in analyzing data during the evaluation of the projects. Unit nursing leadership and staff partnership was invaluable for the success of the projects and for the affirmation of EBP within the unit where the changes have been implemented.

CHANGE IN OPEN VISITATION PRACTICE
Background

In the NICU, a nurse-to-nurse bedside report has been the standard practice for shift change report. In 2007, however, throughout the medical center, the bedside report was changed to include the patient and family in the plan of care as a safety strategy. About the same time, the NICU was in the midst of a large reconstruction plan. Previously, the NICU had multiple beds in one large room, and parents were not allowed to be in the unit during report because of concerns related to patient privacy. After reconstruction, the square footage per bed space tripled, and the beds were separated into three rooms or pods. The coincidence of the NICU construction and the hospital bedside report initiative provided the impetus for the Unit Council shared governance members to examine the bedside report process critically and to explore opportunities for improvement. It was the opportune time to consider an open, less restrictive parent/family visitation policy.

Development of a Searchable Question

The Unit Council chair and co-chair were part of the hospital council that was assisting with the development of the educational components for bedside report. The NICU MCO, CNS, and Unit Council chair and co-chair attended all hospital training sessions addressing the implementation of bedside report. Additionally, the Unit Council chair worked with the librarian and CNS to review the literature related to open visitation in NICUs. To target the search for information specific to the NICU, a searchable question was developed: "Would parental satisfaction be improved if open visitation were permitted in the NICU?" The MCO and the CNS met with the Unit Council to outline an action plan for open visitation based on the search findings, allowing parental involvement in shift report and medical rounds.

Literature Review

The review of the literature showed that the needs of the family must be considered during visitation. The concept of family-centered care in the 1980s first identified family members as care partners.[11] Family-centered care is defined as including families in patient care during medical rounds as well as in the shift report. Including the family in the report provides them an opportunity for education as well as involvement in the patient's care.[12] Inviting the family to participate as a care partner also fosters a trusting relationship between the nurse and family.[13] Family-centered care can be enhanced by using an unrestricted, open visitation policy. Visitation for families who have infants in the NICU needs to be structured for the family, and not the staff.

Ward[14] studied the perception of family needs by surveying parents of infants in a NICU. Using the NICU Family Needs Inventory, Ward found that being able to visit any time was ranked within the top five of the most important needs of these parents. In another study, the amount of visitation in a NICU was correlated with infant and family demographics.[15] The babies with a greater number of hospital days with visitors were more likely to be brought for follow-up appointments than babies with greater number of no-visitor days.[15] Franck and Spencer[16] measured the length of visitation time and the type of activities conducted by mothers and fathers visiting 110 infants in the NICU. Visitation patterns showed the average amount of parental time spent at the bedside was about 2 hours.[16] These findings suggest that visiting meets an important need for parents and also improves outcomes for the infant.

Involving families in shift report and medical rounds allows the parents to feel valued and increases their satisfaction with the health care facility.[17] Ward[14] found that parents' greatest needs were to know exactly what was being done for their infant and to have questions answered honestly. Open visitation is one way to allow parents to identify the best time to visit their infant to see what care is being provided. If parents feel comfortable with the staff, they may want to spend more time at the bedside with their infant, and their presence can generate good communication and have beneficial effects on the infants' outcome.[13]

Evidence also suggests that nursing attitudes toward open visitation may not be positive. Nurses who are comfortable with the status quo may find it difficult to challenge and change an existing practice.[18] Nurses have been opposed to open visitation for three reasons: (1) nurses have varying levels of comfort performing their work with parents at the bedside, (2) nurses believe that parents will be at the bedside continuously and interfere with patient care, and (3) nurses believe that open visitation may lead to the disclosure of sensitive information.[18] Kowalski and colleagues[19] found that 63% of interviewed nurses reported relief when parents were not present during change of shift activities, suggesting that open visitation practices should allow for breaks for parents and nurses, support nurses' judgment of the practice, and maintain confidentiality.

Implementation

A combination of information was used to design the open visitation practice change, including the hospital education materials for improved bedside reporting and the evidence in support of open visitation. The Unit Council modified the hospital education materials for the open visitation changes in the NICU. The material included (1) role playing for social parenting issues that indicated the need for a discussion to occur away from the bedside; (2) positive comments regarding the oncoming nurse so parents felt comfortable with the shift transition; (3) a script to seek permission to include the parents and any additional visitors, if desired, in daily medical rounds; and (4) when it was appropriate to ask visitors to leave. The Unit Council members used the research to persuade staff who were not supportive of the practice change. The members of the Unit Council divided the staff to provide individual education for every staff member. The education included information about the changes to the visitation practices, role playing of anticipated problems, and notification of the date when the unrestricted visitation practice would start.

In addition to the nursing staff, the neonatologists were involved in the open visitation practice change. Initially, the Unit Council chairs met with the physicians to discuss the change for visitation and the educational plan for staff. Then, the unit nursing leadership met with the interdisciplinary team (neonatologists, pharmacy, dietary, chaplain, social work, and other areas) to inform them of the project progress and to discuss any questions. The entire group was receptive to the concept of open visitation, and the neonatologists believed that having parents available to participate in their child's rounds would be helpful for their communication with the parents.

Evaluation

The success of open visitation in the NICU was evaluated using quantitative and qualitative methods. Initially the plan was to obtain feedback using the Press Ganey patient satisfaction survey, but not enough surveys were returned to provide an adequate amount of reporting data. Therefore using the information from the literature, a 12-item satisfaction survey with a five-point Likert scale ranging from very poor to very good was developed to measure parents' satisfaction with the care in the NICU (**Table 1**). The survey was mailed to all families of discharged infants with a postage-paid return envelope. Surveys were returned to a central hospital location where results were tabulated and sent to the NICU MCO. Survey results showed the reaction to open visitation was overwhelmingly positive. Before the institution of open visitation, the patient satisfaction surveys frequently included negative comments about the visitation hours and how parents were kept out of the unit during procedures and medical rounds and at shift change. Since the implementation of open visitation, the parent satisfaction survey results have been extremely positive. From February to May 2008, 100% of parents who responded (n = 29) strongly agreed that it was easy to visit their infant in the NICU.

Additional feedback has been received through communication with parents and open-ended comments on the satisfaction survey. Parents who had experienced the NICU before open visitation noted the improvement in the visitation practice and commented on how it made the NICU more family friendly. The MCO now receives calls from families at other health care facilities asking if they can transfer their baby to this NICU because the family wants open visitation. Actual comments from parents on the satisfaction surveys confirm the positive effect of the change. One response stated: "The doctors and nurses were fabulous! Everyone we came in contact with was friendly, helpful, and supportive. Also, the constant communication was great and helped ease our worries! We also liked the 24/7 visiting hours."

The open visitation practice has been a huge success and has been a source of satisfaction for NICU parents. In addition, the staff has found the change to be positive. Because nurses spend less time addressing parental concerns related to visitation, they have been able to focus on other patient-satisfaction initiatives, such as teaching kangaroo care, guiding parents to create scrap books, and assessing feeding readiness.

CHANGE IN FEEDING READINESS PRACTICE
Background

One of the many challenges premature infants must master before discharge is successful oral feeding. This process might sound like a simple one, because full-term

Table 1 Neonatial ICU parent survey					
Component of Care	**Very Poor**	**Poor**	**Fair**	**Good**	**Very Good**
Care nurses provided to your infant					
Care neonatologists provided for your infant					
Care given to your infant by respiratory therapy, physical therapy, occupational therapy, speech therapy, lactation consultants, and other departments.					
Comfort measures and pain relief provided for your baby					
Nurses and physicians kept you up to date and informed about your infant's progress					
Support, assistance, and privacy were provided for you to breastfeed, care for, or kangaroo your infant					
Ease of visiting the baby					
Opportunity to participate in planning for and providing care for your baby					
Nursing staff provided information and education on your infant's condition(s) and health care needs					
Friendliness/courtesy of the nurses					
Discharge classes prepared you for taking your baby home					
Would recommend Advocate Christ Medical Center/Hope Children's Hospital to a family member or friend					
What most impressed you					
Suggestions for improvement					

newborns usually feed orally with the bottle or breast immediately after birth. Oral feeding, however, requires various skills and reflexes that are still immature in the preterm infant.

Once the onset diagnosis and any other disease process that brought the preterm infant into the unit is resolved, the infant can be categorized as a stable patient or a "feeder-grower" patient. It is now the infant's job to feed, gain weight, and prepare for discharge, not easy tasks to master. Specifically, the infant must learn to suck, swallow, and breathe (SSB) in sequence, without or with minimal drops in heart rate and oxygen desaturations.

Transitioning to oral feedings for the preterm infant requires the caregiver to measure and assess the infant's feeding readiness. Two staff nurses who attended a local conference were introduced to an evidence-based approach for using the infant's behavioral cues while instituting oral feedings. After returning from the conference and observing the customary practice in the unit, it was clear that the practice of advancing feedings was inconsistent and may not have been based on the best evidence. The leadership support of staff attendance at this conference ultimately led to the development and completion of a yearlong project that resulted in a positive change in patient care practice. Two staff nurses led the project to educate staff about the evidential practice of oral feeding and implemented a practice change in the NICU.

Development of a Searchable Question

The first step of this process was to identify systematically the patient care problem in the NICU. The problem was using proper support and feeding techniques to promote adequate nutrition and growth during the infant's transition to oral feedings. The identification of the patient care problem evolved from the questioning of two staff nurses who saw a discrepancy between what was presented at a conference as current evidence and the actual practice on the patient care unit. Working with the NICU CNS and the medical center nurse researcher, the nurses developed a researchable question: "Do preterm infants whose feedings are advanced based on a feeding protocol, compared with current practice, achieve adequate growth and nutrition and have a decreased length of stay?" Once the question was developed, the staff of the unit, in partnership with the CNS, nurse researcher, and librarian, searched for the evidence to provide guidance for the project.

Literature Review

The appropriate time to discharge a preterm infant home is determined by the competency of oral feedings, but there has not been a standard time to initiate the oral feeding process.[20] In the past, the basis for initiating feeding was determined by postconceptual age, weight, and behavioral characteristics such as being able to suck on a pacifier.[21–23] Medical advances have enabled the survival of infants born at earlier gestational ages; thus oral feedings may be introduced before the SSB sequence is present. Some preterm infants have been able to bottlefeed successfully at an age previously believed too early, because the practice was modified in an attempt to decrease length of stay in the NICU.[21,22]

The synactive theory of development as described by Als[24,25] describes the maturational process of behavioral organization in the preterm infant. The framework of this theory addresses the combination of the physiologic and behavioral systems and the way the infant's maturation works to maintain equilibrium between environmental stressors while coping with physiologic demands. This theory suggests that infants function through the "integrated activity of 3 subsystems; autonomic, motoric, and behavioral states."[24,25]

There are physiologic reasons that oral feeding can safely occur before the presence of SSB. Oral feeding for a preterm infant is a high-acuity task,[20,21,23,26–28] and it can be achieved through repetition[21] and the use of positive opportunities.[22,23] Evidence shows that the nurse's role is crucial for the infant to achieve feeding competence.[20–23] Nurses must recognize the initial state of the infant regarding readiness and understand appropriate interventions if the infant becomes distressed during feedings. Nurses also need to provide proper support for the infant during the feeding, which includes encouraging positive feeding experiences. Therefore, it is imperative for the nurse to understand infant cues to feeding readiness when the infant is transitioning to oral feeding.

Readiness often is described as the readiness to feed from a bottle when it is offered.[22] Several factors can contribute to the infant's readiness. Some of these factors are severity of illness, neurologic maturation, and ability to organize autonomic, motor, and behavioral state systems.[20–22,28,29] Depending on the severity of illness, the oral feeding process can be complicated, and the transition period can be lengthened.[22,29] The premature infant's brain is still developing before 34 weeks' gestation, and immaturity of the brain is an important factor in the lack of SSB coordination that makes oral feeding imsuccessful.[21] Typically sucking-swallowing occurs by 28 weeks' gestation, and SSB coordination begins by 32 to 34 weeks.

Several studies have shown that specific behaviors can be observed in infants who are ready for oral feeding. White-Traut and colleagues[28] used secondary analysis of an observational study to find that feeding efficiency can be predicted by the number of feeding-readiness behaviors (FRBs) that the infant exhibits immediately before the feeding. Kinner and Beachy[30] examined nurses' decisions concerning management of feeding in preterm infants in three metropolitan NICUs. Using a self-report questionnaire, the NICU staff nurses ranked factors indicating feeding readiness, behavioral, physiologic, and physical factors, and factors leading to decreasing or eliminating nipple feeds. Results of the study indicated that 54% of nurses worked in units that had guidelines for initiating nipple feeds, and 96% of nurses stated that their units were flexible when it came to managing schedules.[30] The findings suggest that assessment of FRBs can assist nurses in predicting when the infant is ready to begin oral feedings.

Feeding skills evolve continually, even after discharge. Many mothers have expressed concern and have lost confidence in caring for the infant once they are at home.[26] Another approach in aiding the preterm infant to master oral feeds is to involve the parents early in the neonate's stay so the parents can learn to recognize behavioral cues.[20] A structured tool to assess and document the infant's feeding readiness can be used to measure the ability to maintain autonomic stability, engagement, and motor skills before feeding, during feeding, and after feeding.[22,29] The tool can be used both to monitor the infant's progress and as an educational approach when interacting with parents.[27]

Initial skills in premature infants can change over the course of the feeding and between feedings.[27] The Early Feeding Skills Assessment (EFS)[27] is a 36-item observational measure of feeding skills that can be used to assess feeding readiness from the initiation to maturation of oral feeds. The assessment consists of three sections. Section one assesses the infant's state of alertness, oxygen saturation, and energy level; section two assesses the four critical skills domains needed for feeding; and the final section evaluates the impact of the feeding on the infant's alertness, energy level, and physiologic system.[27] The purpose of using the EFS is to give caregivers an ongoing, systematic way to evaluate the infant's strengths and weaknesses and to create individualized feeding care plans for premature infants in the NICU.

Implementation

The evidence supported the use of FRBs as a guide for advancement to oral feedings. The next steps for the team included the assessment of the staff's current practice beliefs, the development of a thorough educational program, and the integration of a FRBs assessment instrument into the standard care processes of the NICU. Because the team aimed to measure patient outcomes to evaluate the effectiveness of the change and hoped to share the results outside the organization, the project protocol, surveys, and methods were approved by the organization's IRB. The CNS and nurse researcher encouraged the team to submit this project to the IRB. By completing the IRB application, the team gained experience about the research process and writing skills needed to develop the literature review. In addition, two surveys were used during the implementation of the project, the EFS[27] and the Oral Feeding Survey.[31] The staff took responsibility for contacting the authors of the tools and asking permission to use their instruments. The authors of the surveys were very willing to share their surveys and personal experience.

To understand the baseline staff knowledge of evidence related to feeding readiness, the Oral Feeding Survey[31] was distributed to the entire staff. The Oral Feeding Survey was designed to measure the criteria that staff use to evaluate whether to initiate or advance to oral feedings in preterm infants. The survey includes nine questions with 34 items identifying cues to begin (eg, observed sucking, strong gag reflex), advance (eg, coordination of SSB, physiologic stability), or decrease (eg, fatigue, poor sucking) oral feedings.

The staff respondents included 117 registered nurses, 18 patient care associates, and seven neonatologists, a 48% response rate from the entire staff. Descriptive analysis of the survey items showed that only 60% of the staff considered behavioral cues when beginning oral feedings (**Fig. 1**). Much of the staff used traditional cues when making decisions to begin oral feedings (**Fig. 2**). Based on the results of the survey and the support of the evidence for change, a standardized educational feeding program was designed to emphasize the use of FRBs, consistent oral feeding techniques, the use of a common language between caregivers, and discharge teaching for parents. The material provided in the teaching sessions included a brief synopsis on the physical growth of the infant, the infant's behavioral cues, and the new feeding protocol. The feeding protocol included a standard feeding assessment schedule,

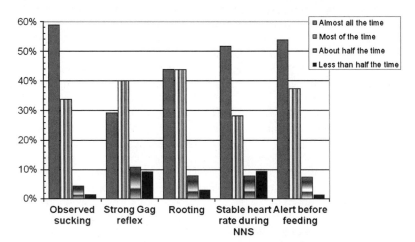

Fig. 1. Criteria for beginning oral feedings: behavioral cues. NNS, non nutritive sucking.

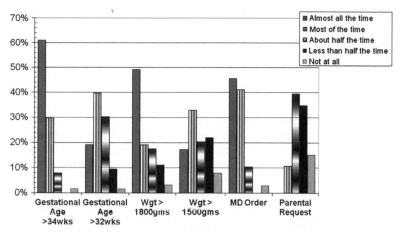

Fig. 2. Criteria for beginning oral feedings: traditional cues. MD, physician.

practice techniques for successful feeding, and educational strategies for parents. Mandatory teaching sessions were provided to the staff of the NICU. To accommodate all the nurses, the session was offered 16 different times over 3 months.

All attendees of the educational sessions were invited to take a pretest and a posttest. A total of 132 staff, including nurses, physicians, speech pathologists, and occupational/physical therapists, attended the education. Once the educational sessions were completed, the feeding protocol and EFS assessment instrument were integrated into the NICU documentation system. Nurses were instructed to use the assessment of FRBs consistently as a guide for assessing the infant's readiness to begin oral feedings. The EFS assessment tool was modified into a chart (**Box 1**) for the nurses to use as a checklist at the bedside. The feeding chart was and continues to be used as a reminder of infants' FRB cues and as a record of an infant's feeding patterns and physical reactions to each feeding, such as decreased heart rate, desaturations, and interventions. Nurses use the assessment data to notify doctors of the infant's readiness and to discuss the proper feeding order for the infant. With the education from the training courses and collaboration with the physicians to write orders according to the feeding protocol, the nurse has the autonomy to increase the oral feeding times based on the infant's FRBs and tolerance of previous feedings.

Box 1
Selected infant feeding assessment criteria
Engagement/readiness cues/feeding skills
Disengagement/distress cues/feeding difficulties
Interventions
Method of feeding
Amount taken/method
Total amount of feeding
Length of oral feeding (minutes)
Fed by parent/nurse

Physicians have been cooperative in implementing the feeding protocol for advancing the infant to oral feedings. The staff nurses are eager to remind the physicians to use the feeding protocol. Evidence that the change is evolving has been found in the orders written by physicians that now read "nipple per feeding protocol" instead of the previous order of "nipple BID" or "nipple 2 to 1."

Evaluation

The pretests and posttests suggested that a need for additional educational reinforcement could be anticipated. It has been approximately 5 months since the last teaching session. Informal evaluation of the change in practice occurred through visual assessment by the unit nursing leadership. Based on the evaluation of the staff's use of the EFS, additional education has been provided on an "as needed" basis. Formal evaluation has begun with a currently ongoing collection of infant length-of-stay data before and after the implementation of the practice change. In addition, the educational session posttest has been incorporated into the semiannual mandatory competencies and will be distributed 6 months after the initial education to assess the staff's level of retention.

The emphasis in this practice change was to shift the feeding paradigm from "volume" to "success." It took time for some nurses and physicians to appreciate the evidence that promoted interactions with the infant for successful feedings not necessarily based on the amount the infant ate. Since the practice change, the staff focuses on making the feeding experience positive so that the infant may continue to feed successfully without tiring and experiencing distress. In addition to the beneficial clinical impact from this practice change, the process of implementing an EBP change was a positive learning experience for the staff and the EBP leaders. The EBP leaders gained personal experience in teaching their colleagues, leading a group through change, and presenting their project at local nursing conferences.

SUMMARY

In a demanding clinical setting, it can be challenging to conduct EBP and follow through with a practice change. In an established Magnet organization that promotes nursing excellence, facilitating the use of EBP is no exception. This Magnet journey allowed the participants to examine the existing nursing research and EBP infrastructure, create positions, establish clean practices, and make improvements that would enable EBP. Early on, the medical center nursing leadership recognized, encouraged, and valued clinical inquiry and change. The chief nurse executive fosters a collaborative environment to deliver evidence-based patient care effectively.

EBP starts with a question, and who is better positioned than the bedside nurse, who lives in the practice environment, to question the day-to-day practices. It is important for nurses to feel supported when questioning practice and to be directed appropriately to translate the project into reality. Both EBP examples described demonstrate that with mentoring and facilitation passionate nurses can succeed in changing practice by using their skills and ability.

Consistent communication and awareness between the facilitator roles is critical so that the appropriate handoffs between the CNS and nurse researcher occur and maintain the project momentum. At the same time, nursing unit leadership needs to continue to provide staff support, time, and resources based on the phase of the project. When EBP project stories are shared with staff, the excitement becomes contagious, and the EBP program can grow, develop, and mature, reducing the gap between practice and research.

One never knows the potential of an EBP project. The benefits can affect individual practice, the organization, and reach as far as local, regional, national, and international practice. Where will your EBP project lead you?

REFERENCES

1. Funk SG, Champagne MT, Wiese RA, et al. BARRIERS: the barriers to research utilization scale. Appl Nurs Res 1991;4(1):39–45.
2. Hutchinson AM, Johnston L. Bridging the divide: a survey of nurses' opinions regarding barriers to, and facilitators of, research utilization in the practice setting. J Clin Nurs 2004;13(3):304–15.
3. Hutchinson AM, Johnston L. Beyond the BARRIERS scale: commonly reported barriers to research use. J Nurs Adm 2006;36(4):189–99.
4. Karkos B, Peters K. A Magnet community hospital: fewer barriers to nursing research utilization. J Nurs Adm 2006;36(7–8):377–82.
5. Melnyk BM, Fineout-Overholt E. Evidence-based practice in nursing & healthcare: a guide to best practice. Philadelphia: Lippincott Williams & WIlkins; 2005.
6. Kitson A, Harvey G, McCormack B. Enabling the implementation of evidence based practice: a conceptual framework. Qual Health Care 1998;7(3):149–58.
7. Rycroft-Malone J, Harvey G, Seers K, et al. An exploration of the factors that influence the implementation of evidence into practice. J Clin Nurs 2004;13(8): 913–24.
8. McCormack B, Kitson A, Harvey G, et al. Getting evidence into practice: the meaning of 'context'. J Adv Nurs 2002;38(1):94–104.
9. Harvey G, Loftus-Hills A, Rycroft-Malone J, et al. Getting evidence into practice: the role and function of facilitation. J Adv Nurs 2002;37(6):577–88.
10. National Association of Clinical Nurse Specialists Statement on clinical nurse specialist practice and education. 2nd edition. Harrisburg (PA): National Association of Clinical Nurse Specialists; 2004. p. 96.
11. Thomas LM. The changing role of parents in neonatal care: a historical review. Neonatal Netw 2008;27(2):91–100.
12. Griffin T. Facing challenges to family-centered care. I: conflicts over visitation. Pediatr Nurs 2003;29(2):135–7.
13. McGrath JM. Partnerships with families: a foundation to support them in difficult times. J Perinat Neonatal Nurs 2005;19(2):94–6.
14. Ward K. Perceived needs of parents of critically ill infants in a neonatal intensive care unit (NICU). Pediatr Nurs 2001;27(3):281–6.
15. Lewis M, Bendersky M, Koons A, et al. Visitation to a neonatal intensive care unit. Pediatrics 1991;88(4):795–800.
16. Franck LS, Spencer C. Parent visiting and participation in infant caregiving activities in a neonatal unit. Birth 2003;30(1):31–5.
17. Davidson JE, Powers K, Hedayat KM, et al. Clinical practice guidelines for support of the family in the patient-centered intensive care unit: American college of critical care medicine task force 2004–2005. Crit Care Med 2007;35(2):605–22.
18. Griffin T. The visitation policy. Neonatal Netw 1998;17(2):75–6.
19. Kowalski WJ, Lawson ML, Oelberg DG. Parent and nurse perceptions of confidentiality, rounding, and visitation policy in a neonatal intensive care unit. Neonatal Intensive Care 2003;16(3):46–50.
20. Thomas JA. Guidelines for bottle feeding your premature baby. Adv Neonatal Care 2007;7(6):311–8.

21. FernÃ¡ndez DÃaz P, Rosales Valdebenito M. International connections. The transition from tube to nipple in the premature newborn. Newborn Infant Nurs Rev 2007;7(2):114–9.
22. Pickler RH. A model of feeding readiness for preterm infants. Neonatal Intensive Care 2004;17(4):31–6.
23. Shaker CS, Woida AM. An evidence-based approach to nipple feeding in a level III NICU: nurse autonomy, developmental care, and teamwork. Neonatal Netw 2007;26(2):77–83.
24. Als H. Toward a synactive theory of development: promise for the assessment of infant individuality. Infant Ment Health J 1982;3:229–43.
25. Als H. A synactive model of neonatal behavioral organization: framework for the assessment of neurobehavioral development in the premature infant and for support of infants and parents in the neonatal intensive care environment. Phys Occup Ther Pediatr 1986;6(3/4):3–53.
26. Reyna BA, Pickler RH, Thompson A. A descriptive study of mothers' experiences feeding their preterm infants after discharge. Adv Neonatal Care 2006;6(6): 333–40.
27. Thoyre SM, Shaker CS, Pridham KF. The early feeding skills assessment for preterm infants. Neonatal Netw 2005;24(3):7–16.
28. White-Traut RC, Berbaum ML, Lessen B, et al. Feeding readiness in preterm infants: the relationship between preterm behavioral state and feeding readiness behaviors and efficiency during transition from gavage to oral feeding. MCN Am J Matern Child Nurs 2005;30(1):52–9.
29. Ludwig SM. Oral feeding and the late preterm infant. Newborn Infant Nurs Rev 2007;7(2):72–5.
30. Kinneer MD, Beachy P. Nipple feeding premature infants in the neonatal intensive-care unit: factors and decisions. J Obstet Gynecol Neonatal Nurs 1994; 23(2):105–12.
31. Scotland J. The regional oral feeding protocol. Calgary, Canada: Calgary Health Region; 2004. p. 1–22.

From the Bedside to the Boardroom: Resuscitating the Use of Nursing Research

Carol Mulvenon, MS, RN-BC, AOCN[a],*, M. Kathleen Brewer, PhD, ARNP, BC[b]

KEYWORDS
- Clinical scholar model • Nursing research
- Clinical research • Implementing nursing research

It is impossible to pick up a nursing journal today and not find at least one article that mentions the importance of research. Providing care that has some science behind it just makes sense. Walk through a hospital in any community today and ask nurses about nursing research, and you probably will get a wide variety of responses ranging from "I don't understand research articles" to "I am a bedside nurse; I have no time for research." In that group of responses, one hopes, there will be a nurse who can describe a practice change based on research that has led to improved patient outcomes. One of the hallmark features of a profession has been described as "how its practitioners use knowledge to make a difference."[1] How then can one persuade the nurse who does not believe she needs to use or do research to move into the professional role of a nurse—one who not only uses existing knowledge but continues to expand the field by questioning practice and searching for answers? This task is not easy. Here is the story of how one organization is accomplishing this goal, one small step at a time.

A BRIEF HISTORY OF RESEARCH WITHIN THE ORGANIZATION

A nursing research committee was started at St. Joseph Medical Center, Carondelet Health System, in Kansas City, Missouri, in 2001. Membership consisted of four advanced-practice nurses and several motivated staff nurses who participated when they could get someone to cover their patient assignment on the floor. A purpose statement was developed, and the functions of the committee were described. It was determined that the promotion of evidence-based practice would

[a] Pain Management, Palliative Care, Oncology, St. Joseph Medical Center, Kansas City, MO 64114, USA
[b] University of Kansas School of Nursing, 3901 Rainbow Boulevard, Kansas City, KS 66160, USA
* Corresponding author. 4138 Blackjack Oak Drive, Lawrence, KS 66047.
E-mail address: cmulvenon@carondelet.com (C. Mulvenon).

Nurs Clin N Am 44 (2009) 145–152
doi:10.1016/j.cnur.2008.10.006
0029-6465/08/$ – see front matter © 2009 Elsevier Inc. All rights reserved.

underpin nursing practice. The committee members also recognized the importance of educating nurses about how to use and conduct research. Within months of the committee's formation, an issue surfaced regarding the way blood pressure was taken. What better way to promote research and educate nurses than by conducting a study?

The agony of a good idea gone awry will not be described in detail. The limited research experience of the group quickly became evident. The investigation was begun before the question was completely defined. Operating from a quality improvement mindset, approval from an institutional review board was not obtained. Armed with enthusiasm and a problem clearly needing to be addressed, the group set out to assess baseline data, review the evidence, and make recommendations for change based on evidential findings. Valuable knowledge for the organization was obtained from this "study." Changes were made in how blood pressures were assessed. New equipment was purchased. Alas, this knowledge could not be shared with the broader nursing community because it was more of a quality improvement project than a formal study. Help was needed from an experienced researcher. For a period of time the committee collaborated with a local school of nursing, and a doctorally prepared nurse attended meetings. This informal relationship was vitally important in getting started, but it was evident that more structure was required and that a formal arrangement with a nurse researcher must be established.

As the committee struggled to find its way with the process of conducting research, education was provided for staff members about nursing research. The goal of this education was to emphasize why the practice should be guided by evidence and not based on the traditional views of the most outspoken nurse at the meeting. Attendance at educational programs was small and erratic. Nurses at all levels of practice continued to express feelings of intimidation regarding conducting research and using it to inform their practice. Frustration among the committee members mounted. Eye rolling was seen, and deep sighs were heard before, during, and after meetings. In Shared Leadership councils, policies were updated dutifully on a regular basis using the most current reference from the literature. No, the resources were not always evidence based, but they were published in journals.

Steps were being taken, the committee had been formed, a study had been undertaken, education was occurring, but the goal of promoting evidence-based practice was not being achieved at a desirable level. In retrospect it is easy to see that there was not a clear vision of what was to be achieved. "Promotion of research and the use of evidence" is not as specific as "nurses actively questioning their practice and becoming knowledgeable about how to find answers that are supported by evidence." This lack of direction made it impossible to plan and achieve what was desired. The same education process continued: a reiteration of what research is and why it is important. Unsurprisingly, nurses were not engaged with this approach.

Despite the lack of a clear vision and a plan, some key components were in place. From the outset, there was complete support from nursing administration. All clinical nurse specialists had research incorporated into their job descriptions. Nursing research and quality improvement was an integral part of the career advancement program. There was access to literature through the hospital library, and a skilled, approachable librarian served as an excellent resource for literature searches and obtaining articles as needed. There were computers in the clinical nurse specialists' offices as well as on all nursing units, and access to the Internet was available. Nursing research was included explicitly in the budget of the organization. One change that occurred in this time frame was the expansion of the committee to include nurses not from just one institution, but from two, encompassing all the nurses within the

organization. This expansion created a few logistical challenges, but, more importantly, the research committee members still felt that something vital was lacking.

RESUSCITATING THE VISION

If this were a fairy tale, we would tell you that one day the nursing research committee
awakened and proclaimed "Enough of this time-wasting stuff that has gone on for the
last 5 years. From this day forth, nurses within the organization will stop thinking that
evidence-based practice means updating the reference list of policies and will begin to
question practice actively and to learn a method through which practice can be
changed. Everyone will like it and participate!" Oh no, enlightenment did not come
like that. What did occur, though, was a case of excellent timing. The two integral
components of a vital plan—a vision and a reliable process—somehow came together
at just the right moment.

The vice president of nursing had heard about the Clinical Scholar Model at a training
session that she attended to be come a new Magnet program appraiser.[2,3] The pre-
senters reported a winning formula for bringing the bedside nurse and research together in a large tertiary care hospital, with a nurse researcher as coordinator and
facilitator of the program. Could an organization without a full-time researcher
realistically implement a similar program? The presenter, who had initiated this
point-of-care program, was invited as a keynote speaker to talk with the direct care
nursing staff about research at the bedside and with managers about their role in
creating the environment that would support this research. "We want nurses to see
that research is important and something they can do," we told her. "We want you
to put on your super hero cape and swoop down among the nurses and sprinkle fairy
dust and get them fired up about research." Those may not have been the exact
words, but that is what we wanted to ask for. This was a tall order, much to ask of
a speaker who was coming in for 1 day and visiting each institution for 2 hours. But
she did it. She used examples to which nurses could relate. She shared stories
from the hospital where she worked, with research and evidence-based practice examples that resonated with the nursing staff. She made the program seem like something we could do. More than that, she somehow made staff nurses realize that
nursing research was not stuffy and impossibly hard. Instead she made it relative.
She used language that nurses understand. Attendance at the programs was high.
Nurses remarked in their evaluations that they had "not gotten the connection"
between research and practice before, but after hearing this presentation they did.
The members of the nursing research committee saw a glimmer of hope. A clear vision
had been provided.

The Clinical Scholar Model was selected as the foundation for how a nurse might
evaluate and possibly change practice.[3] Once the model was selected, various
institutions that had adopted the model were studied to determine how they had
developed nurses in the role of clinical scholars. The goal was to determine how the
nursing department at Carondelet Health system could individualize the model to
work within both institutions using the current available resources. Simultaneously,
the search was ongoing for a part-time nurse researcher. Time was a big factor.
The program needed to be implemented while nurses still were enthusiastic about engaging in research.

The nursing research committee discussed putting together an education program
for the nurses who would participate in the Clinical Scholar Program. But what would
be the most effective way to prepare nurses to evaluate existing practices critically?
The committee met. They discussed the issues. What should be included in the

education for staff? Who should teach the classes? How would staff be mentored through the process? Merely providing a blueprint for transitioning from staff nurse to clinical scholar would not provide the support needed to sustain nurses through the pitfalls and frustrations that would arise in their investigations.

A search was conducted to find templates and educational material that had been used in other facilities to increase the conduct and use of research by point-of-care providers. A continuing education program was located on the Sigma Theta Tau International website (www.nursingknowledge.org). Instead of re-inventing the wheel, should we use this program? We contacted our speaker, because she had offered to provide additional consultation. Could this program work in our organization? She advised us, "try one and see what you think." How very sensible. A copy was purchased and completed. All the essential elements required in conducting a review of the literature and determining whether to make practice changes or conduct further research were included. A decision was made to use this curriculum, and it was purchased by the organization for all participants in the Clinical Scholar Program.

Around the time the decision to use the online program was made, a nurse researcher applied to the organization and was hired. At last, a voice of experience was available to provide direction and expertise when needed. The actualization of our vision was in sight.

FULFILLING THE VISION

Armed with clear vision (ie, that nurses would question their practice actively and would be knowledgeable about how to find answers that are supported by evidence), a reliable process (ie, the Clinical Scholar Program), and a ready guide (ie, our nurse researcher), we set out on our journey. An application was developed and sent to all the nurses in the organization, encouraging them to be a part of the Clinical Scholar Program. Most of the nursing research committee members made a commitment to participate in the online Clinical Scholar Program as well. There was discussion at the meetings about the number of nurses to enroll in the program. The enrollment of one or two nurses from every unit, or at least one or two nurses from every clinical area, would result in a very large number of participants. A suggestion was made to actively recruit individuals who were considered to be ready for this type of challenge. Others thought it might be best to start small and simply select individuals who applied for the program, rather than actively trying to recruit. Members of the committee would be involved actively in an investigation of their own. Although most committee members had conducted some research in the past, none thought they were experts. Could they actively assist a number of uncertain recruits while conducting their own investigation? After a thorough discussion, it was decided to keep the numbers small and to select nurses who were motivated and confident enough to submit an application on their own. Depending on the outcome of the first group of scholars, this program would continue in the future with increasing participation from nurses throughout the organization.

Nurses were selected for the program based on the merits of their completed application and the endorsement of their manager. With the guidance of the nurse researcher, the clinical scholar group would select issues to investigate and carry out the steps of the research process as they completed each part of the online program. In a group setting, participants would discuss and problem solve barriers they encountered in their quests to implement evidence-based practice.

The plan was for the education of the clinical scholars to unfold over a 3- to 5-month period, culminating with the annual nursing research fair to showcase work accomplished by clinical scholars as they worked to make evidence a tangible, meaningful part of everyday practice.

A DIARY OF THE CHALLENGES AND SUCCESSES
January 10, 2008

Applications have been reviewed, and the clinical scholars have been selected. A total of 10 individuals, including members of the nursing research committee, will participate in the program. Participants include five staff nurses, three clinical nurse specialists, a nursing administrator, and the nurse researcher. The plan is to have a poster forum this summer to showcase the work of the clinical scholars.

I am very glad to be moving beyond this never-ending cycle of trying to explain what research is and how we are supposed to be or are using it. I am ready to begin conducting investigations into issues so that we can show people better by doing things. I think most nurses learn best when they have an example they can see.

February 14, 2008

After a few snags all the participants in the clinical scholars program have been able to sign in and have begun the program. Time was spent discussing briefly what topics each participant may want to delve into deeper. Three members of the group are fairly certain about their topic. Six members have a vague idea or are trying to decide between two topics.

One of our members has dropped out of the program. She passed her materials on to another nurse at her facility. I will need to evaluate if he will be a good candidate for this program and be certain of his commitment. I am disappointed that we have already lost one of our staff nurse members and someone that I thought would be good in this role, but I am glad that she dropped out now instead of later after she had already started part of the program. I know there are likely to be more dropouts. I am not sure how you can prevent it. I thought I did a pretty good job of making clear what the expectations were and did not try to talk anyone into undertaking this program, knowing that it would be difficult to keep people in the program with all the other directions they are being pulled in. Today a blackboard or angel site for the research committee to use was discussed. I am excited about the ability for the participants in the program to communicate with each other in this way at their convenience. Time is always a big issue, and having everyone meet at the same time is hard.

March 13, 2008

The nurse researcher demonstrated the angel site that will be available for communicating informally among the group between meetings. Some have used this form of communication in school; others do not yet have a clear picture of how it will work but express a desire to be able to communicate electronically when they have the time. There was good discussion about three of the clinical scholars' topics.

A staff nurse from the operating room (OR) is interested in exploring the lack of a written record of the physician orders during the intraoperative period and the possible impact on the patient from a safety perspective. Potential ramifications discussed include the potential for duplicate orders or omissions in care. The discussion included steps that would be needed to get this information on the chart, what staff members in the OR think about this issue, and what the benefits of this change would be. Suggestions were provided regarding directions for a literature search and an investigation of the community standard.

The reduction of nursings' footprint in pharmaceutical waste is the topic a staff nurse in the ICU is exploring. Discussion centered on how and to what extent nurses contribute to the problem. The group is unsure of the process currently used by pharmacy to dispose of waste. A variety of ways that nurses can impact the issue were discussed, including educating patients about disposal of medications.

Open visitation in the postanesthesia care unit (PACU) has been of interest to a nurse from this department since she went to a national conference several years ago and heard about a hospital that allowed it. Benefits included very high levels of satisfaction from patients. This nurse is concerned about studying this topic because open visitation in the current physical environment of the PACU could infringe on patient privacy. There are mixed feelings about this issue among the nurses in the recovery room as well. Suggestions were made regarding a review of the available literature regarding ICU and pediatric visiting hours.

Unfortunately not everyone had a chance to discuss their topic. Next month the meeting will occur via a teleconference between our two facilities. I am concerned about the possible impact on discussion and the ability to communicate easily. All the clinical scholars have completed module one. A new staff nurse has replaced the one who was unable to continue. It is good to have a researcher here to assist with the development of individual questions and to focus more precisely on the issues. Keeping the group on target can be challenging. We only have 1 hour each month in which we get together formally to talk about this program. I struggle with the issue of making the meetings longer, but my experience tells me that longer meetings generally lead to more time wasting.

April 10, 2008

Today the meeting started with a discussion of the projects being considered by the members of the group who did not share last month.

An emergency department nurse who also is a clinical instructor has selected a topic regarding preceptors and their needs when precepting a student. She is working with a fellow instructor on this study, and they are applying for a clinical research grant. They have reached the point of seeking approval for this study from the Human Subjects Committee at the university. This study also will need to go to the Research Steering Committee at the hospital.

The orientation of patients as they are transported is the subject of interest to an ICU nurse. She wants to know if there is any validity to transporting a patient feet first. She reports that studies done regarding this practice have been conducted on healthy people. A member of the group mentioned reviewing research done comparing amounts of antiemetics used with patients who were loaded feet first or head first into medical evacuation helicopters.

The director of nursing in the clinical scholars group is exploring family-initiated rapid assessment team calls. She reports not finding research published on this topic. There are recommendations regarding the need for this practice in the literature, but no studies or guidelines exist. The group suggested looking at available literature on the topics of family presence in codes or family involvement in patient care. Evaluating material presented at conferences that may not yet be in literature also was discussed.

One of the clinical nurse specialists is focusing on early indicators of dehydration in the patient. Her focus is on early identification by the nurse and interventions to improve patient outcomes.

Another topic proposed is the co-administration of blood and opioids administered via a patient-controlled analgesia (PCA) pump. Blood bank standards and hospital policy generally do not allow the simultaneous administration of blood with any other products except normal saline. This prohibition can lead to poor pain control or the need for another intravenous site to continue the PCA. A search is underway to determine the rationale for this prohibition and the data that support the practice.

We are discussing ideas in real, not theoretic, circumstances. It feels different. Instead of talking but knowing no change will take place, we are appraising situations critically. It feels empowering instead of frustrating. The exchange of ideas among the group is invigorating. A call for abstracts has been received for the 11th Kansas Nursing Research Exchange. Can anyone be ready to submit an abstract by the deadline called for? Our nurse researcher assures us that we can. Writing abstracts remains a bit intimidating to those of us who have not done much of it. It's a good thing we have someone to encourage and help us.

May 8, 2008

Work progresses on the refinement of the questions at the heart of each clinical scholar's investigation. The study on preceptors' needs has been submitted to the Human Subjects Review Board and is awaiting word on approval. The review of literature for the pharmaceutical waste study has been completed. The next step is development of a survey with the help of our researcher.

The operating room nurse has become frustrated with her topic because she cannot find anything in the literature, but her enthusiasm for the program remains undampened. She has decided to tackle her initial topic of physician's orders in the OR from a quality improvement perspective and to work on the importance of normothermia in the perioperative patient for the Clinical Scholars Program. A committee member suggested a review of what is happening with normothermia in military hospitals. This milieu also was suggested as a resource for the issue of co-administration of blood and opioids.

The issue of open visiting hours in the postanesthesia care unit has become overwhelming for the nurse who wants to make this change happen. She reports that she does not know where to focus and feels that she will meet resistance no matter what she does. The nurse researcher helps her to focus on just one aspect of the issue—surveying the nurses in the department about reasons to allow visitors in the area and reasons not to let visitors in.

Another clinical nurse specialist reported on her topic of the prevention of deep vein thrombosis (DVT). Despite safety initiatives and efforts by hospitals aimed at preventing DVTs, some patients still develop them. Treatment in the acute phase focuses on anticoagulation and prevention of pulmonary embolism. These patients also are at risk for long-term complications, such as postthrombotic syndrome, venous insufficiency, and venous stasis ulcers, that can be extremely debilitating. The use of compression therapy following a DVT has been shown to reduce the incidence and severity of long-term complications, but most patients either are never counseled to wear them or choose not to comply. She plans to explore the reasons why patients do not use compression therapy after an acute DVT.

As work progresses among the clinical scholars, you can feel the excitement of the group. Although challenges have arisen, the group members remain engaged in the process. Chairing this committee has moved beyond the drudgery of research hanging around my neck like a ball and chain to feeling good about knowing the resources are there and we actually are in the process of undertaking investigations and doing it right. We are still working on the use of the angel site. I think it will be a good method of communication between our meetings. It seems hard to get what we need to get done in an hour, but everyone has other commitments as well.

WHERE WE ARE TODAY

Since the nursing research committee began to meet approximately 7 years ago, we have learned some tough lessons. Is it necessary and perhaps even helpful to go through the trial-and-error process to be where we are today? For those who subscribe to the "no pain—no gain" way of thinking, maybe it is. We like to think we are more enlightened than that. What rescued our nursing research committee from certain death was the coming together of the vision, a plan, and a ready resource. It helped immensely to have someone come to our organization and show us that what we wanted to do was possible. Seeing an example of how someone had accomplished it enabled us to believe we could, as well. Along with the vision, the Clinical Scholars Program is turning out to be a reliable roadmap. This structured approach for teaching nurses the steps needed to conduct an investigation the proper way feels right for us. The third and absolutely essential piece of our success is the nurse researcher who serves as our guide and mentor, encouraging us along the way and providing the expertise and support we need as we continue to grow and develop.

The group has committed to complete the Clinical Scholars curriculum by the summer of 2008. Several have completed it already and are moving full steam ahead on their projects. The decision to start with a small group of clinical scholars was a good one for us. A larger group would have made it very difficult to give each topic the time and attention warranted. We are just at the beginning of our journey, with much yet to accomplish. As our organization continues on the path of achieving our vision for research, this current group of clinical scholars will be able to mentor the next group and broaden the base of support for nursing research, one clinical scholar at a time.

REFERENCES

1. Hegyvary ST. To make a difference. J Nurs Scholarsh 2007;39(1):1–2.
2. Schultz AA. Nursing research, research utilization, evidence-based practice. Houston (TX): New Magnet Appraiser Workshop; 2007.
3. Schultz AA. Clinical scholars at the bedside: an EBP mentorship model for today. ENK: Excellence in Nursing Knowledge 2005.

Index

Note: Page numbers of article titles are in **boldface** type.

A

Academic medical centers, application of evidence-based practice model in, **1–10**
 case study, 7–9
 developing the program, 2–7
  academic program, 5–7
  clinical program, 3–5
Analysis, of evidence-based practice, and critique, in model for staff nurses, 14
 example of, in Clinical Scholar model, 101
Application, of evidence-based practice, example of, in Clinical Scholar model, 101
 in model for staff nurses, 14
Assessment, of evidence, to incorporate into policies and procedures, 57–58

B

Barnes-Jewish Hospital, Evidence Equals Excellence program at, **1–10**
Baylor Health Care System Professional Nursing Practice Model, staff nurses creating safe
 passage with, 73–80
  engaging nurses in evidence-based practice, 74–76
  linking nursing evidence and patient outcomes, 76–80
Bedrest, optimal length of, following cardiac catheterization or percutaneous coronary
 intervention, Clinical Scholar model in evaluation of, 117–122
Best practices, nursing quality program driven by evidence-based practice, **83–91**
 Best Practices Council, 84
 St. Luke's Evidence Based Practice Model, 84–86
 using or implementing best practice model, 86–89
  bloodstream infection prevention, 87
  fall prevention, 87–88
  hands-off communication, 88–89
  pressure ulcer prevention, 88
Bloodstream infections, prevention of, implementing best practices for, 87

C

Cardiac catheterization, reducing length of bed rest following, use of Clinical Scholar model
 in evaluation of, 117–122
Cardiology nursing, evidence-based practice in, improving glycemic control in open-heart
 surgery program, 124–128
 reducing length of bed rest following cardiac catheterization or percutaneous coronary
  intervention, 117–122
 reducing postoperative nausea and vomiting in patients undergoing open-heart surgery,
  122–124

doi:10.1016/S0029-6465(08)00097-2
0029-6465/08/$ – see front matter © 2009 Elsevier Inc. All rights reserved.
nursing.theclinics.com

Children's hospitals, experience with evidence-based practice model in, 20–24
Clinical nurse specialist (CNS), role of, in evidence-based practice, 133–134
Clinical practice. *See* Evidence-based practice.
Clinical Scholar Program, development and implementation of, **93–102**
    clinical exemplar: policy for oral fluids prior to patient discharge, 100–102
        analyzing, 101
        applying and evaluating, 101
        disseminating, 101
        observing, 100–101
        synthesizing, 101
    cultural readiness, 94
    definition of evidence-based practice, 93–94
    development of the model, 94–96
    implementation of, 96–98
    sustaining the model, 99–100
    the model, 96
        description, 96
        essential components of, 96
        goals, 96
    who is the clinical scholar, 98–99
  embracing evidence-based practice in a rural state, **33–42**
  in community hospitals, **11–25**
    development of model, 12–13
    experience at a community hospital, 15–20
    experience at a freestanding pediatric hospital, 20–24
  resuscitation of nursing research with, **145–152**
  three evidence-based projects using the model, **117–130**
    improving glycemic control in open-heart surgery program, 124–128
    reducing length of bed rest following cardiac catheterization or percutaneous coronary intervention, 117–122
    reducing postoperative nausea and vomiting in patients undergoing open-heart surgery, 122–124
Collaboration, among urban hospitals through Texas Christian University Center for Evidence-Based Practice and Research, **27–31**
  Maine Nursing Practice Consortium, **33–42**
Communication, hands-off, implementing best practices for, 88–89
Community hospitals, building capacity for research and evidence-based practice in, **11–25**
    Clinical Scholar Program, 13–14
      experience at a community hospital, 15–20
      experience at a freestanding pediatric hospital, 20–24
    development of clinical scholar model, 12–13

D

Design, of policies and procedures incorporating evidence-based practice, 59–63
Dissemination, of evidence-based practice findings, example of, in Clinical Scholar model, 101
  in model for staff nurses, 14
DVDs, preoperative instructional, effects on patient knowledge and preparedness, **103–115**

E

Education, nursing, application of evidence-based practice model in academic medical center, **1–10**
case study, 7–9
developing the program, 2–7
academic program, 5–7
clinical program, 3–5
National Quality Forum Scholars Initiative for practicing nurses, **43–55**
Education, patient, preoperative instructional DVD on postoperative care activities, **103–115**
discussion, 112–114
evidence-based literature, 104–107
intervention for project implementation, 107–108
postintervention results, 108–112
purpose of project, 107
scope of problem in existing practice, 104
Evidence Equals Excellence (EEE) program, in an academic medical center, **1–10**
case study, 7–9
developing the program, 2–7
academic program, 5–7
clinical program, 3–5
Evidence-based practice, 1–152
building capacity for, in staff nurses, **93–102**
clinical scholar model for, **117–130**
collaboration among urban hospitals for, **27–31**
health system-wide educational program for nurses in, **43–55**
in a rural state, **33–42**
in an academic medical center, **1–10**
in community hospitals, **11–25**
nursing quality program driven by, **83–91**
patient education with preoperative instructional digital video disc, **103–115**
promoting safe outcomes in, **57–70**
resuscitating use of nursing research, **145–152**
staff nurses creating safe passage with, **71–81**
to improve care for vulnerable neonatal population, **131–144**

F

Fall prevention, implementing best practices for, 87–88
Feeding readiness, in neonatal intensive care unit, evidence-based changes in practice, 136–142
Fluids, oral, prior to patient discharge, evidence-based practice resulting in policy change, 100–102
analyzing, 101
applying and evaluating, 101
disseminating, 101
observing, 100–101
synthesizing, 101

G

Glycemic control, improvement of in open-heart surgery program, 124–128

H

Hands-off communication, implementing best practices for, 88–89
Hospitals, academic medical centers. *See* Academic medical centers.
    community. *See* Community hospitals.
    urban. *See* Urban hospitals.

I

Implementation, of policies and procedures incorporating evidence-based practice, 63–69
Infections, bloodstream, prevention of, implementing best practices for, 87
Informatics, in National Quality Forum Scholars Initiative for practicing nurses, **43–55**
Integration, of policies and procedures incorporating evidence-based practice, 69

J

John C. Lincoln North Mountain Hospital, experience with Clinical Scholar program at,
    15–20

L

Leadership, development of, in National Quality Forum Scholars Initiative for practicing
    nurses, 49
Linking, of evidence to outcomes, to incorporate evidence into policies and procedures,
    58–59

M

Maine Medical Center, development of Clinical Scholar program at, 12–13, **93–102**
    three examples of staff nurses' projects using the Clinical Scholar model at, **117–130**
Maine Nursing Practice Consortium, embracing evidence-based practice in a rural state
    through, **33–42**
        lessons learned, 40–41
        Maine Nursing Practice Consortium, 37–38
            first year accomplishments, 38–39
        outcomes of workshops, 40
        process of solidifying a collaborative partnership, 36
        workshop on promoting evidence-based practice through a spirit of inquiry, 36–37
        workshop on renewing the spirit of nursing, 39–40
Mayo Clinic, National Quality Forum Scholars Initiative for nurses at, **43–55**
Mentoring, in an evidence-based practice model in an academic medical center, **1–10**
Mentorship, development of, in National Quality Forum Scholars Initiative for practicing
    nurses, 49
Models, Baylor Health Care System Professional Nursing Practice Model, 73–80
    Clinical Scholar Program, at St. Joseph's Medical Center, Kansas City, 147–149
        development of, **93–102**
        in community hospitals, **11–25**

three examples of staff nurses' projects using the, **117–130**
use to promote evidence-based practice in a rural state, 34–36
Evidence Equals Excellence program, **1–10**
National Quality Forum Scholars Initiative for practicing nurses, **43–55**
Promoting Action on Research Implementation in Health Services (PARHIS) framework,
    71–73
St. Luke's Evidence Based Practice Model, 84–86

N

National Quality Forum Scholars Initiative, implementation by Mayo Clinic Nursing, **43–55**
    case examples from evidence-based practice project teams, 48–49
    challenges in, 49–51
    facilitating factors, 51–52
    intended participants, 46
    leadership and mentorship in, 49
    lessons learned, 52
    program description, 45
    program implementation, 46–48
    specific program goals, 46
    summer assignment (Appendix), 53–54
Nausea, postoperative, reduction of in patients undergoing open-heart surgery, use of
    Clinical Scholar model in evaluation of, 122–124
Neonatal intensive care nursing, using evidence to improve care in, **131–144**
    change in feeding readiness practice, 136–142
    change in open visitation practice, 134–136
    clinical nursing research, 132–133
    role of clinical nurse specialist, 133–134
    role of professional nurse researchers, 133
Nurse researcher, professional. *See* Researcher, professional nurse.
Nurses, staff. *See* Staff nurses.
Nursing education. *See* Education, nursing.
Nursing research. *See* Research, nursing.

O

Observation, example of, in Clinical Scholar model, 100–101
    reflection and, in evidence-based practice model for staff nurses, 13–14
Open-heart surgery, evidence-based practice in, improving glycemic control in patients
    undergoing, 124–128
    reducing postoperative nausea and vomiting in patients undergoing, 122–124
Oral fluids, *see* Fluids, oral.
Outcomes. *See also* Safety, patient.
incorporating evidence into policies and procedures for promotion of safe, **57–70**
    assess, 57–58
    design, 59–63
    implementation, 63–69
    integrate and maintain, 69
    link, 58–59
    synthesis, 59

P

Partnerships, among urban hospitals through Texas Christian University Center
    for Evidence-Based Practice and Research, **27–31**
Patient education. *See* Education, patient.
Patient safety. *See* Safety, patient.
Pediatric hospitals, experience with evidence-based practice model in, 20–24
Percutaneous coronary intervention, reducing length of bed rest following, use of Clinical
    Scholar model in evaluation of, 117–122
Phoenix Children's Hospital, experience with Clinical Scholar program at, 20–24
Policies, procedures and, incorporating evidence into, for promotion of safe outcomes,
    57–70
        assess, 57–58
        design, 59–63
        implementation, 63–69
        integrate and maintain, 69
        link, 58–59
        synthesis, 59
Postoperative care activities, effects of preoperative instructional DVD on patient
    knowledge and preparedness for, **103–115**
        discussion, 112–114
        evidence-based literature, 104–107
        intervention for project implementation, 107–108
        postintervention results, 108–112
        purpose of project, 107
        scope of problem in existing practice, 104
Postoperative nausea and vomiting, reduction of in patients undergoing open-heart
    surgery, use of Clinical Scholar model in evaluation of, 122–124
Preoperative instructions, effects of preoperative instructional DVD on patient knowledge
    and preparedness, **103–115**
Pressure ulcers, focus on, by evidence-based practice project teams in National Quality
    Forum Scholars Initiative, 48–49
prevention of, implementing best practices for, 88
Procedures, *see* Policies, procedures and.
Professional development, in National Quality Forum Scholars Initiative for practicing
    nurses, **43–55**
Promoting Action on Research Implementation in Health Services (PARHIS), 71–73

Q

Quality, nursing, program for, driven by evidence-based practice, **83–91**
        Best Practices Council, 84
        St. Luke's Evidence Based Practice Model, 84–86
        using or implementing best practice model, 86–89
            bloodstream infection prevention, 87
            fall prevention, 87–88
            hands-off communication, 88–89
            pressure ulcer prevention, 88

R

Reflection, observation and, in evidence-based practice model for staff nurses, 13–14

Research, nursing, building capacity for in community hospitals, **11–25**
    clinical, in neonatal intensive care unit nursing, 132–133
        role of clinical nurse specialist, 133–134
        role of professional nurse researcher, 133
    collaboration in, among urban hospitals through Texas Christian University Center for
        Evidence-Based Practice and Research, **27–31**
    resuscitating the use of, from bedside to boardroom, **145–152**
        brief history of research at St. Joseph's Medical Center, Kansas City, 145–147
        challenges and successes in, 149–151
        fulfilling the vision for, 148–149
        vision for, Clinical Scholar Model in, 147–148
        where we are today, 152
Researcher, professional nurse, role of, in evidence-based practice, 133
Rural areas, embracing evidence-based practice in, **33–42**
        lessons learned, 40–41
        Maine Nursing Practice Consortium, 37–38
            first year accomplishments, 38–39
        outcomes of workshops, 40
        process of solidifying a collaborative partnership, 36
        workshop on promoting evidence-based practice through a spirit of inquiry, 36–37
        workshop on renewing the spirit of nursing, 39–40

S

Safety, patient, incorporating evidence into policies and procedures, **57–70**
        assess, 57–58
        design, 59–63
        implementation, 63–69
        integrate and maintain, 69
        link, 58–59
        synthesis, 59
    staff nurses creating safe passage with evidence-based practice, **71–81**
        Baylor Health Care System Professional Nursing Practice Model, 73–80
            engaging nurses in evidence-based practice, 74–76
            linking nursing evidence and patient outcomes, 76–80
        creating urgency for, 72
        factors influencing implementation of, 72–73
St. Joseph's Medical Center, Kansas City, resuscitating the use of nursing research at,
    145–152
        brief history of research at, 145–147
        challenges and successes in, 149–151
        fulfilling the vision for, 148–149
        vision for, Clinical Scholar Model in, 147–148
        where we are today, 152
St. Luke's Hospital, Houston, Best Practices Council for nursing quality at, **83–91**
Staff nurses, evidence-based practice by, 1–152
        building capacity for, **93–102**
        clinical scholar model for, **117–130**
        collaboration among urban hospitals for, **27–31**
        creating safe passage with, **71–81**
        health system-wide educational program for, **43–55**

in a rural state, **33–42**
in an academic medical center, **1–10**
in community hospitals, **11–25**
nursing quality program driven by, **83–91**
patient education with preoperative instructional digital video disc, **103–115**
promoting safe outcomes in, **57–70**
resuscitating use of nursing research, **145–152**
to improve care for vulnerable neonatal population, **131–144**
Surgical patients, cardiology, evidence-based nursing practice in, improving glycemic control in open-heart surgery program, 124–128
 reducing length of bed rest following cardiac catheterization or percutaneous coronary intervention, 117–122
 reducing postoperative nausea and vomiting in patients undergoing open-heart surgery, 122–124
effects of preoperative instructional DVD on patient knowledge and preparedness, **103–115**
 discussion, 112–114
 evidence-based literature, 104–107
 intervention for project implementation, 107–108
 postintervention results, 108–112
 purpose of project, 107
 scope of problem in existing practice, 104
Synthesis, of evidence, example of, in Clinical Scholar model, 101
in evidence-based practice model for staff nurses, 14
to incorporate evidence into policies and procedures, 59

T

Texas Christian University Center for Evidence-Based Practice and Research, **27–31**

U

Urban hospitals, development of evidence-based practice and research collaborative among, **27–31**
 activities, 28–29
 challenges, 29
 future goals, 31
 hospital perspective, 30
 successes, 30–31

V

Visitation, parental, in neonatal intensive care unit, evidence-based changes in practice, 134–136
Vomiting, postoperative, reduction of in patients undergoing open-heart surgery, use of Clinical Scholar model in evaluation of, 122–124

Moving?

Make sure your subscription moves with you!

To notify us of your new address, find your **Clinics Account Number** (located on your mailing label above your name), and contact customer service at:

E-mail: elspcs@elsevier.com

800-654-2452 (subscribers in the U.S. & Canada)
314-453-7041 (subscribers outside of the U.S. & Canada)

Fax number: 314-523-5170

Elsevier Periodicals Customer Service
11830 Westline Industrial Drive
St. Louis, MO 63146

*To ensure uninterrupted delivery of your subscription, please notify us at least 4 weeks in advance of move.